P9-CIU-735

01323658

RC 537 .M65 1990
Depression : the mood
Mondimore, Francis Mark
disease   132365

DATE DUE

DATE DUE

FEB 22 1996	APR 2 8 1997	FEB - 2 1999
SEP 25 1996	JUL 2 4 1997	MAY 1 0 1999
OCT - 8 1996	OCT 1 6 1997	FEB - 4 2000
OCT 22 1996	DEC - 3 1997	
NOV - 4 1996	FEB - 1 1998	
NOV 1 8 1996	MAR 27 1998	FEB - 2 2001
DEC 1 9 1996	SEP 2 5 1998	MAR 0 1 2002
DEC 3 0 1996	Oct 8 1998	
FEB 1 0 1997		
24	NOV 2 4 1998	NOV 1 9 2003
APR - 7 1997	MAR 2 0	

MAR 3 0 1993	
SEP 2 3 1993	APR 1 0 1995
OCT - 5 1993	
OCT 2 1 1993	OCT 1 5 1995
	OCT 3 0 1995
NOV 6 1993	NOV 1 3 1995
DEC - 7 1993	DEC - 1 1995

BRODART, INC.   Cat. No. 23-221

DEPRESSION, THE MOOD DISEASE

D E P R E

OKANAGAN COLLEGE LIBRARY
BRITISH COLUMBIA

S S I O N

THE MOOD DISEASE

Francis Mark Mondimore, M.D.

THE JOHNS HOPKINS UNIVERSITY PRESS
BALTIMORE AND LONDON

© 1990 The Johns Hopkins University Press
All rights reserved
Printed in the United States of America

The Johns Hopkins University Press
701 West 40th Street, Baltimore, Maryland 21211
The Johns Hopkins Press Ltd., London

Library of Congress Cataloging-in-Publication Data

Mondimore, Francis Mark, 1953–
  Depression, the mood disease / Francis Mark Mondimore.
     p.   cm.
  Bibliography: p.
  Includes index.
  ISBN 0-8018-3856-8 (alk. paper)
  1. Depression, Mental—Popular works. I. Title.
RC537.M65 1990
616.85′27—dc20   89-34654
                                            CIP

*The paper used in this publication meets the minimum requirements of
American national standard for Information Sciences—Permanence of Paper
for Printed Library Materials, ANSI Z39.48–1984.*

To J. R., friend and companion

CONTENTS

Preface   ix

Notes on Sources   xiii

PART ONE **SYMPTOMS, DIAGNOSIS, AND TREATMENT**

1. Mood   3

    Mood: What Is It?   3 ▪ *The Chemistry of Mood*   6 ▪ *The Mood Disorders*   11

2. Depression   15

    The Depression of Affective Disorder   15 ▪ *The Symptoms of Major Depression*   23 ▪ *Other Types of Depression*   27 ▪ *The Classification of Depression*   31

3. Treatment   42

    The Treatment of Major Depression   42 ▪ *Complicated Depression*   66 ▪ *Tests for Affective Disorder*   75

4. Bipolar Disorder   79

    "Manic-Depressive Illness"   79 ▪ *"Mood Swings" and Cyclothymia*   87 ▪ *The Chemistry of Bipolar Disorder*   90 ▪

The Treatment of Bipolar Disorder   92 ▪ *Length of Treatment in Bipolar Disorder*   101

PART TWO **VARIATIONS, CAUSES, AND CONNECTIONS**

5. Variations of the Mood Disorders   107

Major Depression in the Elderly   108 ▪ *Mood Disorders in Children and Adolescents*   113 ▪ *Mood Disorders in Women*   117 ▪ *Depression and Stroke*   126 ▪ *Depression and Pain*   130 ▪ *Seasonal Affective Disorder*   136 ▪ *Schizoaffective Disorder*   142 ▪ *Panic Attacks and Mood Disorders*   144

6. Causal Factors and Associations   152

The Heredity of Mood Disorders   152 ▪ *Drug and Alcohol Abuse and Mood Disorders*   156 ▪ *Medical Causes of Mood Disorders*   163 ▪ *Sleep and Depression*   170

PART THREE **GETTING BETTER**

7. Advice for Mood Disorder Patients and Their Families   177

Who Can Help? The Mental Health Professionals   178 ▪ *Living with a Mood Disorder*   185 ▪ *Psychotherapy*   200 ▪ *Psychiatric Hospitalization*   205 ▪ *Stigma*   211

8. Summing Up   214

Further Reading   219

Index   221

PREFACE

Depression, "mood swings," and other mood disorders are estimated to afflict up to 15 percent of the adult population at any given time. Even though safe and effective treatments for this group of illnesses are readily available, study after study has concluded that many, perhaps most, of the people who suffer from them do not receive adequate treatment. This book is for these people and their families.

Every year hundreds of thousands of people are given prescriptions for antidepressant medications but stop taking them because they never receive a thorough explanation of their purpose or side effects and are not carefully instructed in how to take them properly or in what kinds of improvement to expect and how soon. This book is for them.

Uncountable thousands seek relief for their mood problems from family members, counselors, and clergy when they actually suffer from a medical illness and need to see a physician. Perhaps many more simply suffer in silence, not knowing what to do or whom to ask for help. Most of all, this book is for them.

This is not a "self-help" book. Perhaps it is closer in style and content to a "consumer's guide." My purpose is to explain that in many cases a mood disorder such as depression is a serious medical problem. It is not something one can talk oneself out of, not a "phase of life problem," not "getting old," "growing pains," or some other minor and temporary difficulty that will pass with time or that people can "snap out of." It is a medical illness that causes lost productivity and time off from work at a tremendous dollar cost. It brings great misery: wasted days, months, and even years of impaired functioning at a human cost that cannot be measured. It is a disease with a frightening mortality rate. Its most serious complication, suicide, often takes its victims in the prime of life and is consistently one of the top ten causes of death at all ages. Suicide is the third leading cause of death in teenagers and young adults. Nevertheless, these illnesses are misdiagnosed by doctors, misunderstood by many well-educated laypeople, and, tragically, too often ignored or explained away as a passing inconvenience.

I have written this book to help people with depression and other mood disorders understand their illness and their treatment so they can get the fullest benefit from all available types of therapy.

In these first paragraphs, you may have noticed some words that are perhaps unexpected: *disease, illness, complications, mortality rate.* These are "medical" words, not "psychological" words, used in discussing diseases of the body like tuberculosis, myocardial infarction (heart attack), or diabetes. I hope that by the time you have finished this book you will agree that they are completely appropriate for discussing mood disorders and that depression or abnormal mood swings can be as much a disorder of the body as any other "real" disease you can think of.

I recommend you read the book from beginning to end in sequence. The beginning chapters lay some important groundwork for those that come later. Also, don't assume that some of the "special case" sections (such as "Depression and Stroke" in chapter 5) don't apply to you and therefore be tempted to skip them. Many facts learned by studying special cases have shed light on all the mood disorders. Scientists have learned much from them, and so will you.

If you bought this book to understand your own feelings of depression, your mood swings, or the "moody" behavior of someone close to you, that in itself probably points to a medically treatable mood disorder. I think you will find this volume informative and comforting, but don't think it can substitute for medical treatment! Remember, it is a consumer's guide, not a repair manual. Read the book *and* make an appointment to see your doctor. Today.

I want to acknowledge many sources of help and inspiration

for this book. Dr. Paul McHugh, chairman of the Psychiatry Department and the Henry Phipps Professor of Psychiatry at Johns Hopkins University, taught me that psychiatry is real medicine and real science. He also taught me that the best clinical teachers are patients and that I must listen to them carefully. Dr. J. Raymond DePaulo, associate professor in psychiatry at Johns Hopkins, taught me that mood disorders are the most misunderstood and misdiagnosed illnesses in psychiatry—perhaps in all of medicine. I also want to thank the staff of the Community Psychiatry Program of the Francis Scott Key Medical Center in Baltimore, especially Wayne Swartz, for support, for encouragement, and for teaching me that dedication and commitment are the most important parts of being in one of the helping professions.

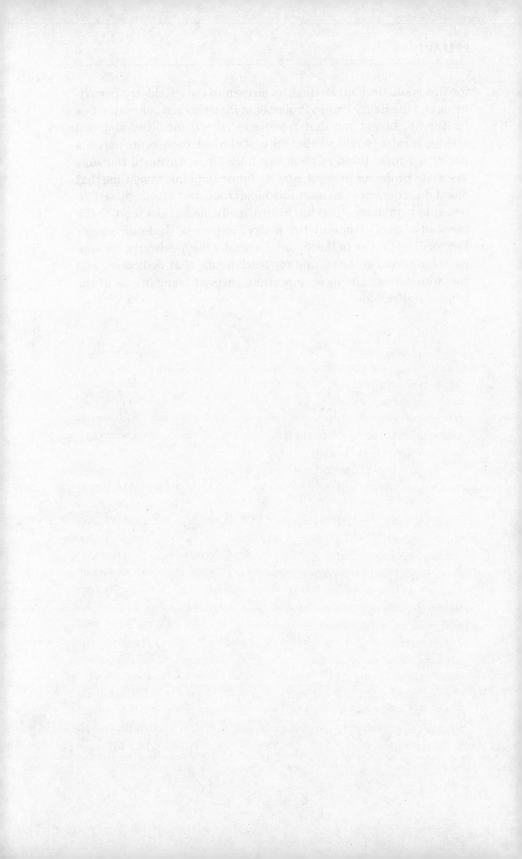

NOTE ON SOURCES

Because I have written this book for anyone afflicted or concerned with affective disorders, I have not distracted lay readers with references according to the standards usually applied to scientific and scholarly works. Nonetheless, a general comment on the sources for my material is in order.

I have tried to adhere to the clinical classifications and diagnostic criteria of the *Diagnostic and Statistical Manual of Mental Disorders*, third edition, revised (DSM-III-R) of the American Psychiatric Association (Washington, D.C.: American Psychiatric Association Press, 1987) in my discussions of symptoms and signs of the various mood disorders. In describing treatments, I have taken as current standards of practice the approaches and recommendations of standard textbooks in psychiatry such as *The Comprehensive Textbook of Psychiatry*, fourth edition, edited by Kaplan and Saddock (Baltimore: Williams and Wilkins, 1985). Other textbook and review sources were the *American Psychiatric Association Annual Review*, volume 6 (Washington, D.C.: American Psychiatric Association Press, 1987) and Hollister's *Clinical Pharmacology of Psychotherapeutic Drugs*, second edition (New York: Churchill Livingstone, 1983). Much material was also derived from review articles in clinical psychiatric journals such as *Psychiatric Annals* and the

Journal of Clinical Psychiatry. Most valuable have been the peer-reviewed psychiatric journals of the American Psychiatric Association *(American Journal of Psychiatry)* and the American Medical Association *(Archives of General Psychiatry).*

PART ONE

Symptoms, Diagnosis, and Treatment

ONE

MOOD

Mood: What Is It?

"I'm in a great mood today; I feel on top of the world." "Stay out of my way this morning, I'm in a terrible mood." We use the word *mood* all the time to describe a complicated set of feelings, both psychological and physical, that affect our behavior toward others, our productivity, our ability to relax and have fun, and our attitude about ourselves.

When our mood is good we feel energetic, optimistic about the future, and eager for the challenges of work or play. In a good mood, we are outgoing and enjoy being with people. We have a hearty appetite, sleep soundly through the night, and awake refreshed and ready for a new day. People in a good mood are affectionate and loving, and sex is relaxed and fun. Perhaps the most basic aspect of a good mood is that it makes us confident—sure of our positive attributes and not preoccupied by our faults. Minor setbacks are taken in stride, and even major problems can be tackled with determination and commitment. A person in a good mood is happy to be alive.

A bad mood causes an opposite set of feelings. The half-filled glass looks half empty. Energy is low, and it's hard to get things done—the most minor tasks seem interminable or even overwhelming. Time passes slowly. In a bad mood we find other people irritating and may lose our temper over the smallest things, then feel guilty for having done so. Not surprisingly, we simply avoid others and prefer to be alone. It's difficult to be affectionate and almost impossible to be sexy. More basic is a feeling of emptiness, of not being our usual self; self-confidence is absent, self-esteem low. This is the set of changes and feelings psychiatrists call *depression*.

Unfortunately, discussions of mood states and changes in mood have suffered from a lack of precise medical terms to describe them. This has hampered medicine's ability to discuss mood problems in a way that is as precise and therefore, to some people's way of thinking, as "medical" as, say, a discussion of headaches or chest pains. But it's not easy to discuss such very basic and complex feelings the same way one talks about a physical pain. A physical pain can usually be described very precisely. One can often point to a location on the body, rate the pain in intensity, and say when it began. "It hurts more when I cough"; "I've got a throbbing headache." These are symptoms that can be characterized very accurately.

Doctors have always had a hard time naming symptoms that are more generalized and difficult to pinpoint, so this trouble in describing mood is not surprising. To describe how one feels when the flu is coming on, the aching in muscles and joints, hot and cold feelings, headache, and so forth, English-speaking physicians merely borrow the French word for illness and call this collection of symptoms *malaise*. It's not surprising, then, that we have not come up with good terminology for the symptoms of the disease that affects mood. Mood is such a basic aspect of how one feels that it is difficult to describe it, talk about it precisely, or identify mood changes within oneself or others in specific terms. In questioning patients, psychiatrists often resort to slang. A good mood is referred to as "on a high," "in high spirits." A bad or low mood is referred to as "down in the dumps," "in low spirits," "the blues."

So what is meant by the commonly used word *depression*? Many people say "I'm depressed" when they really mean "I'm sad." *Depression* does not really mean *sadness*. Usually a person feels sad about something in particular, and the feeling is usually associated with some loss. For example, people become sad about the death of a loved one or the breakup of a relationship. Other words used to describe this sense of loss are *grief* and *bereavement*. Another kind of sadness is the sense of longing for the way things were, for the "good old days," that is commonly called *nostalgia*.

Unfortunately, the word *depression* is often inaccurately used to describe these other unpleasant feelings. The concept as psychiatrists use it is a bit different, a more fundamental and also more pervasive experience. Sometimes depression can go far beyond sadness and the other feelings described above to affect the way we feel about our entire future and alter some very basic attitudes about ourselves. Sometimes depression can deepen and widen to poison one's attitude about all aspects of life, to the point where words like *despair* and *hopelessness* accurately reflect one's feelings. Another word used to separate this collection of feelings from other sad feelings is *melancholia*. This very old word means "black bile" and refers to the ancient Greek theory of medicine that considered disease states to be caused by a deficiency or excess of one of four bodily fluids. (Depressed persons were thought to suffer from an excess of black bile.) Although *melancholia* was the word used to describe depression in several very early clinical works on psychiatric conditions and thus might seem a natural choice as a modern clinical term, it has never gained common acceptance, perhaps because of its poetic, romanticized connotations.

I hope this discussion helps you begin to understand what psychiatrists mean by mood. Yes, it does include concepts like happy and sad, but mood goes further or perhaps deeper than this and includes our sense of physical well-being, our attitudes toward others, our feelings about the future, our self-esteem and confidence, and our attitude toward ourselves as well.

What is a *normal* mood? It would be easy to get into a complicated philosophical and scientific discussion on the question What is normal? To keep things simple, I will use the word *normal* to mean that which is usual, common, or expected—not some ideal state against which other states or conditions are compared.

Let's get back to the question, What is a normal mood? The first part of the answer is, it depends. A good mood is frequently normal, but a bad mood can be normal as well. For example, when good things happen to us, we generally find ourselves in a good mood. When we are beset by problems, disappointments, and setbacks, it is normal to be in a bad mood. The "it depends" part is perhaps one of the most important characteristics of normal mood, for normally mood is *reactive*. Our mood responds and reacts to events—to what happens to us and to those important to us. Furthermore, mood is reactive in a predictable way: when something good happens, our mood is good; when something bad happens, our mood turns sour. Thus a second aspect of normal mood is that the direction of changes in mood is *understandable* in light of what we know about human nature and the way people usually react to events.

Another characteristic of normal mood changes is that they are in some way *proportional* to the circumstances that provoke them. For example, the normal change in mood following the death of a spouse will be very severe, much more than following the death of a pet. Getting a big promotion would be expected to lead to a greater boost in mood than merely being let off early one afternoon. Everyone has an intuitive sense of the direction and degree of mood change to be expected in particular circumstances; our sense is based on our own experience and observations. Although psychiatrists have been trained to observe people closely and are experienced in judging the usual range or proportion of mood change, we too rely quite a bit on intuition in drawing conclusions about normal and abnormal moods.

So it's not so much the mood state itself that can be said to be abnormal. More important, really, is to see the mood in the context of life events. Again, normal mood is reactive to life events, the way it changes is understandable in light of those events, and the change is proportional to the events.

The Chemistry of Mood

One of the greatest revolutions in medicine occurred during the seventeenth and eighteenth centuries when physicians began to realize that the workings of the human body followed the rules of science. Indeed, the word *science* came to be used in its modern sense during this time and replaced the older term *natural philosophy*. Today we take for granted that the heart is a pump and that we can understand a lot about the way it works if we know how pumps work. After the Frenchman Pouseille described the laws of physics that determine the flow rate, pressure, and other properties of fluids flowing through glass tubes, it quickly became apparent that the flow of blood through arteries and veins followed the same principles. "Philosophical" speculations on the heart as the source of love, loyalty, and other poetic qualities and feelings disappeared and were replaced by cold, hard, usually mathematical rules and principles.

You may be wondering, What does this have to do with mood? Isn't this aspect of the human experience above the laws of science or at least beyond them? Well, in the past fifteen years or so another scientific revolution has been going on. It's a quiet revolution, and only those who read medical and scientific journals are even aware of it. This quiet revolution is taking place in the fields of neuroscience (the study of the brain and nervous system) and psychiatry (the branch of medicine that concerns itself with treating disorders of emotions and behavior). What we are learning today is that the activities of the human brain—activities like thinking, remembering, getting angry, and feeling calm—can also be understood in scientific terms and follow the laws of biology and chemistry.

This application of the laws of science, especially biochemistry (the chemistry of living things), to understanding and predicting behavior and mental states isn't really surprising or even new. Man has known for thousands of years that various chemicals can change thinking and behavior. Almost as soon as we figured out how to grow crops, we discovered how to ferment some of them and began using ethyl alcohol (the alcohol in alcoholic beverages) to change the way we feel. We found substances that dull the perception of pain (aspirin from the bark of willows, morphine from poppies), substances that boost mood and energy level (for example, coca leaves, the source of cocaine), and other substances that could induce very abnormal mental experiences such as hallucinations (peyote cactus buttons, the source of mescaline, for example). The number of naturally occurring psychoactive substances has now been far surpassed by man-made ones, and the list goes on and on. (*Psychoactive* means having an effect on the activities of the brain and on mental processes.)

As more and more chemicals were discovered and used as medicines to treat everything from tuberculosis to arthritis, many of these were found to be psychoactive as well. Important to our topic was the discovery in the 1950s that reserpine, used to treat high blood pressure, caused profound depression in some people. People who had been pefectly happy became suidical while taking this medication. This was one of the first pieces of evidence that there is a chemical basis to mood, and it is still one of the most compelling.

The Workings of the Nervous System

To understand the chemistry of mood, we must know a little about how the nervous system works. Although the details are very complicated, there are a few basic principles that are not difficult to grasp.

The nervous system, including its most important organ, the brain, is like a large collection of electrical wires. Nerve fibers carry electrical signals along their length, signals that can be measured with sophisticated equipment but that are very low in voltage. In some places the "wires" are stretched out and travel great distances. The long nerve that travels from the spinal cord to the tip of the big toe is like the telephone wires you see stretching along a country road. Some "wires" are extremely short but connect to many others. This arrangement is seen in the largest part of the nervous system, the brain. The organization inside the brain is more like the organized tangle of wires in a phone company relay box.

The big difference between the circuitry of the telephone system and that of the nervous system is that in the nervous system the end of one "wire" does not connect to the tip of the next. There is a microscopic space between one nerve cell and the next. A chemical messenger carries the signal across this space; this messenger is called a neurotransmitter. The complete process of signal transmission in the nervous system, then, consists of the electrical signal traveling along a nerve fiber to a terminal point, where it causes packets of the neurotransmitter chemical to be released. The neurotransmitter flows across the tiny space and by matching up with other chemicals on the surface of the next cell (called receptors) turns on the next cell's electrical system, so that another electrical impulse starts "down the line" (see fig. 1).

The revolution going on in neuroscience is the explosion of information about the neurotransmitters. As it turns out, the electrical activity of each nerve cell is rather simple—each cell is more or less "on" or "off." It is the chemical switches, the neurotransmitters, that are really important. Many neurotransmitters have been discovered, and more and more substances that have been known

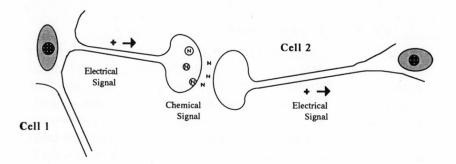

Figure 1   Nervous system signal transmission. N = neurotransmitter molecule

to exist in other organs of the body are being found to have neuro-transmitter functions as well. Some of the more important are dopa-mine, norepinephrine, GABA, and acetylcholine. I'll be discussing them in more detail later.

It may seem odd that in the nervous system, where electrical activity is so prominent, chemical activity is turning out to be even more important. Another rather recent advancement in science, however, makes this finding less surprising. The computer/word processor I used to type this book is made of many, many tiny units, any one of which can only be on or off. It is the changing pattern of "ons" and "offs" that allows the computer to calculate, remember, and so forth. What determines the pattern is a set of many switches.

Another very important fact that has been discovered in neuro-science is that the brain uses particular neurotransmitters to run particular systems—to do certain things. *Dopamine* runs a system that regulates body motion and helps many sets of muscles work together to bring about smooth movements. *Norepinephrine*, among other things, regulates the "fight or flight" response; that is, when this system is activated the heart beats faster, adrenaline is released into the bloodstream, and a state of alertness is produced so that thinking seems clearer and one is ready for quick response. *GABA* seems to tone down the functioning of many different areas of the brain, producing a state of calmness. The anxiety medication di-azepam (Valium) may mimic this neurotransmitter.

Disease and Neurotransmitters

Parkinson's disease is a progressive deterioration of a person's ability to produce smooth muscle movement. The first sign of this devastating disease is usually a change in muscle tone that shows up as stiffness and slowness of movement. A person walks with a shuffle and becomes stooped. The limbs tremble. Writing is scrawled. In severe cases the victim becomes almost paralyzed. These symptoms occur not because the muscles or nerves in the limbs are diseased, but because the organization and initiation of movement in the brain centers controlling these functions fails. Sometimes this failure is so profound and movement becomes so disorganized that the patient is nearly immobolized.

Not so long ago—less than eighty years, in fact—it was discovered that Parkinson's disease is caused by the deterioration of a single brain center, the substantia nigra (literally "black substance," so called because this area appears to the naked eye to have dark pigment). This center was found to be connected to many other areas of the brain that control movement, and it is thought to somehow coordinate all these centers to produce smooth, fluid motion. The chemical messenger of this center is the neurotransmitter dopamine. In fact, the brains of persons who had died with Parkinson's disease were found on autopsy to have much less dopamine than normal in the substantia nigra. It seemed that the loss of dopamine-producing cells somehow upset the balance of activity of brain centers necessary for smooth movement, causing the symptoms of Parkinson's disease.

Under the microscope, many cells of the substantia nigra in people with Parkinson's disease could be seen to be dead or dying. One unfortunate fact about the nervous system is that once nerve cells are dead or injured, they usually do not grow back. (The most familiar example, and one of the most tragic, is spinal cord injury; once the cord is injured, paralysis is permanent.)

But even if the cells were dead and could not grow back, was it possible to replace the chemical the dead cells had once produced? Could the amount of dopamine in the system be somehow boosted back toward the normal level? The answer fortunately is yes. When we administer the drug L-dopa, which the body changes into dopamine, the symptoms of Parkinson's disease often respond dramatically. Increasing the amount of dopamine available to the cells remaining in the substantia nigra restores a more normal balance among the neurotransmitters regulating movement, and this vital function returns toward normal. This was one of the first examples of "neurotransmitter therapy" that developed from an understanding of the chemistry involved both in normal brain functioning and in the disease state. For the first time, neuroscientists figured out the chemistry of a system in the brain and set out to treat a disease by manipulating that system. Also for the first time, they were successful.

The Mood Disorders

I have talked about chemicals that affect emotions and behavior and about how the brain uses chemical messengers called neurotransmitters to carry out its functions. I discussed Parkinson's disease, which is caused by a lack of a particular neurotransmitter and which is treated by boosting the level of the missing chemical in the brain. With these facts in mind, let me pose several questions:

1. Since the brain uses chemical messengers to carry out its work and to regulate things like muscle tone and level of alertness, shouldn't there also be neurotransmitters that regulate mood?

2. Can't we assume that the chemicals that affect mood (like the blood pressure medicine reserpine that causes depression in some people) work by affecting these neurotransmitters?

3. Might there not be a type of disease that affects this set of neurotransmitters and has as its symptom an abnormal change in mood?

4. Couldn't we treat this disease with medication that restores the balance of neurotransmitters to normal?

The answer to all these questions is yes! There is a group of illnesses affecting mood that have been called by many names over the years (and unfortunately still are called by many names) and that are definitely related in some as yet undiscovered way. Some psychiatrists think all these illnesses and their variations are so closely connected that they should be considered subtypes or variations of a single disease, which has been called *affective disorder*. Nevertheless, because the relationship between them is really almost completely unknown, the variations are listed in the official diagnostic manual of the American Psychiatric Association one by one simply as *mood disorders*. Like many psychiatrists, I will use these two terms more or less interchangeably.

The word *affective* has been used for many years by psychologists and psychiatrists to talk about mood. It refers both to the subjective experience (how one feels on the inside) and also to the changes in behavior and functioning that can accompany a marked change in mood (the sad look of a depressed person, loss of appetite, restlessness, and so forth).

Why aren't these illnesses called affective *diseases* or mood diseases? After all, we don't call the movement problem I discussed earlier Parkinson's *disorder*. The answer is that medical scientists are reluctant to call a process a disease if its basic cause is unknown or if we cannot see its basic pathology—abnormalities that can be observed under a microscope or measured in a laboratory. Scientists investigating Parkinson's disease saw deterioration and death of cells in the brains of its victims and measured changes in the amount of dopamine: unequivocal pathological changes.

In affective disorder, the changes are just beginning to be measured. Because they seem to be chemical, there are no changes in the structure of the brain that can be seen with a CAT scan or MRI scan or observed at autopsy. Because the chemical changes appear to be so subtle and because the amounts of brain chemicals are so small and difficult to measure, chemical analysis has not been much help either.

Nevertheless, the indirect evidence is compelling that mood changes sometimes result from an abnormal change in the balance of neurotransmitters in the brain. I chose the title of this book, *Depression, the Mood Disease*, because I want to emphasize that this problem is a medical illness that requires assessment and treatment by a doctor.

What do I mean by indirect evidence? I mentioned earlier that in the 1950s severe depression was noted in some people who took reserpine for high blood pressure. Several years later it was discovered that reserpine seems to work by depleting the amount of the neurotransmitter norepinephrine at the ends of the nerves that go to blood vessels. It was theorized that reserpine must have the same effect somewhere in the brain, in an area or system controlling mood, and that lack of norepinephrine in this other system brought on severe depression. Unfortunately, the simple conclusion that depression is caused by lowering norepinephrine in the brain is not the whole story. First, not all patients who take reserpine get depressed. Second, although some of the medications used to treat depression do boost norepinephrine, others that are equally effective seem to have little effect on this neurotransmitter.

This brings us to a second piece of indirect evidence for a chemical basis of some depression: there are medications that are effective in treating it. Unlike the scientific discoveries and elegant reasoning that led to a treatment for Parkinson's disease, the medications and other treatments used for depression were discovered essentially by accident. It was only after they had been used safely and effectively for some time that some of their effects on brain chemistry were discovered. Again, it was shown that some boost the amount of various neurotransmitters and otherwise seem to affect the functioning of the neurotransmitter systems in the brain.

This evidence is indirect because no one has discovered patterns of neurotransmitter changes that are always seen in particular mood disorders and succeeded in measuring them. You can probably see why. First of all, you can imagine that a brain system regulating a state as basic as mood might not be a small center that is easily pinpointed. It might be more like a network of nerve fibers going to many, many different areas of the brain and coordinating many different functions. Since, as we have seen, change in mood affects appetite, sleep, sexual desire, and so forth, this makes a lot of sense. Second, if no death of cells is involved (unlike Parkinson's disease), looking at brain structure under the microscope will be fruitless. (More detailed discussion of the possible location of a mood-regulating system in the brain will be presented in chapter 5 in the section titled "Depression and Stroke.") Nevertheless this kind of evidence— and more is being discovered every day—points unequivocally to a chemical basis for affective disorder or the mood disorders.

With this background, and the knowledge that abnormalities of mood can result from a change in the chemistry of the brain that requires proper diagnosis and medical treatment, we'll begin our exploration of mood disease. I'll discuss symptoms and treatment for the different types of mood disorders and also, in chapter 5, talk about some cases of mood disorders that require special approaches or have revealed new facts about this mysterious group of illnesses and led to new theories or treatments. We'll pick up lots more information on neurochemistry along the way, and in the last chapter you'll see why psychiatrists are so optimistic that our understanding of mood disorders and our ability to treat them are just beginning.

We'll start with the most common form of mood disorder—and one of the frequent problems any doctor treats—depression.

TWO

DEPRESSION

The Depression of Affective Disorder

There is no more vivid way to talk about a disease and its symptoms and treatment than the case study. Throughout this book, I will use case studies to explain a symptom or make a point. Some of the cases are composites of many patients; all the facts have been altered and disguised to protect the privacy of the people involved.

Margaret was a thirty-two-year-old woman who was referred to me by her family doctor because she was "very depressed." When I first saw her in my office she was attractive and fashionably dressed and looked healthy, but she had a sad, subdued manner.

"Your doctor told me you've been feeling depressed," I said. "How long has this been a problem for you?"

Margaret sighed deeply; she looked as if she didn't know where to begin. "About six months, I guess." Another deep sigh. "The crazy thing is, Doctor, I have absolutely no reason to feel like this. Feeling depressed is not like me."

"You'd better be careful using the word *crazy* in a psychiatrist's office!" I said smiling, trying to be reassuring.

She looked blankly at the picture opposite her chair; if she had

heard my attempt at humor, she certainly didn't think it was
funny.

She continued: "I have a wonderful husband; we have two
healthy children who do well in school and don't cause any problems at home other than the usual brother-sister bickering. No one
could ask for a better family."

Margaret had just returned to full-time work the year before
when her younger child was old enough to be in day care. She was
executive director of the local arts council and had been enjoying
her work immensely until her mood changes began. Margaret was
well educated and had been very successful in her career in the
arts. She had attended a prestigious local women's college and had
a bachelor's degree in English and a master of fine arts degree. She
had held administrative positions in several arts organizations
before she got married and for a time afterward, but she quit
working while her children were infants. While she was at home
after the birth of her second child, she did watercolors in her spare
time. She'd had a show of these works at one of the better galleries
in town two years before and continued to sell her work regularly.

Her husband was an attorney with a medium-size firm and
was well on the way toward becoming a partner. I saw from her
address that they lived in a distinguished older neighborhood—
finances were probably not a problem. Why was this attractive,
healthy, successful young woman depressed?

"Think for a minute about the beginning of this depression.
What was the first thing you noticed that you thought wasn't
right?"

"I think the very first thing I noticed was that I started having
trouble sleeping. I've always slept very soundly."

"I want you to think carefully about your sleep problems for a
moment. Have you been having trouble falling asleep at night, or
do you notice that you wake up early in the morning and can't get
back to sleep?"

"Let me think about that. I just seem to toss and turn all
night, I think." She paused for a moment. "Well no, I know I lie
awake waiting for the sunrise many mornings. I think it's more the
second pattern."

"Do you think about anything in particular in those early
morning hours?"

Another sigh. "Oh, I don't know . . . depressing things; it seems
I obsess about every foolish thing I've ever done in my life."

"Like what?"

She was quiet for a moment and looked across the room at the
picture again. "Well, my husband's sure this is the problem, so I
might as well just tell you right away." (This might explain it, I
thought, she's going to reveal some terrible secret, the basis for her
early morning ruminations and other symptoms of depression.)

Margaret's "terrible secret" was that she had become pregnant
as a teenager and had had an abortion.

"When did your husband find this out?" I asked.

"I told him before we got married."

Well, this doesn't quite fit, I thought. I could have understood if
Margaret's husband had just found out about a prior intimate relationship and had become jealous and accusing, perhaps taunting
her about it or perhaps becoming sullen and withdrawn. Opening
old wounds like this has a way of making a person relive all sorts
of regrets and losses and can definitely cause temporary depression.
But that this successful, talented young woman would suddenly
start worrying about such an old issue didn't quite make sense.

"Has someone else just found this out, or has something else
happened to bring this issue up again? Problems between you and
your parents, perhaps?"

"Not really."

In fact, Margaret's family had been very supportive at the
time of her teenage pregnancy, and she had even received pastoral
counseling before and after the abortion. Her mother had taken
her to the clinic the day of the procedure. It had been a first-
trimester abortion, and no one outside the family had even known
about it. Years later she had decided to tell her fiancé about the
entire episode so it would not be an issue that would ever come
back to bother her.

"Can you think of any reason this should have started troub-
ling you again now?"

"None. I really thought I had dealt with all of that years ago.
It was a chapter in my life that I had just turned the page on."

I tried to find other clues to her symptoms in the content of
her early-morning thoughts. "Tell me what else you find yourself
obsessing about."

"I worry about the children, especially Sarah, my youngest.
I feel I should be at home for her until she's in the first grade like I
was for David." She paused and sighed deeply. She looked down at
the floor and said with a pained voice, "I have had such guilty feelings about her being in day care."

Margaret didn't realize that by using one particular word in
her last sentence, only fifteen minutes into her first appointment
with me, she had allowed me to diagnose the depression of affective disorder and decide on a plan of treatment.

"Do you think there's a connection between your feeling about
Sarah's day care and your memories of the abortion?"

As Margaret looked down at the floor, her mouth began trem-
bling and tears welled up.

"Doctor, I sometimes have these awful guilty feelings that I'm
a terrible mother." She started crying quietly. "I've never felt so
bad in my life."

<hr>

Are you wondering what word made the diagnosis? "Made the
diagnosis" is perhaps overstating the case. Let me say rather that
it is a word that makes a psychiatrist highly suspicious of a mood
disorder in a person complaining of depression. The word is *guilty*.
A peculiar quality of the depressed mood seen in affective disorder
is that it is very often accompanied by feelings of guilt. Sadness,
disappointment, and other unpleasant feelings we discussed earlier do not usually have this quality, whereas patients suffering with
the depression of affective disorder frequently find their thoughts
drifting back to things they have regretted or felt guilty about. Very
often, as in Margaret's case, they feel guilty about things they thought
they had come to terms with, and they can't explain the recurrence
of bad feelings about these old issues. Margaret had shared her
experience with all the important people in her life she felt had
a right to know, even her husband, whom she met years after the
incident had occurred and who might never have found out otherwise. Margaret clearly felt guilty about the abortion now, but she
hadn't for many years. No one in her life had brought it up. Why
were these feelings coming up now?

Many mothers feel a bit guilty initially about sending their children to day care, even now when so many young women work outside

the home. But guilty feelings had not cropped up for Margaret until the past several weeks, and this was many months after the child had started day care. As it turned out, little Sarah had done some clinging when she first started at day care, but in a week she was completely adjusted to the routine, had made lots of friends, and looked forward to going each morning. Again, Margaret's guilty feelings should have been strongest when Sarah was in the clinging stage, not now. Margaret's feelings were not entirely *understandable* in light of the facts of her life situation.

"You've already told me about your sleep problem. Have you lost your appetite?" I asked.

"Yes, most days I just force myself to eat, especially breakfast."

"Have you lost weight?"

"A few pounds, but I can stand to lose a few."

"Have you noticed that you've lost interest in sex?"

"Yes . . . that's really bothering me too. My husband and I have always had such a good relationship, it's not like me not to be interested in him."

The evidence for the depression of affective disorder was accumulating fast; here were the typical *vegetative symptoms*. Vegetative symptoms refer to the symptoms that the depression of affective disorder causes because it interferes with the basic needs or drives for sleep, food, and sexual pleasure. That this illness interferes with so many aspects of life illustrates how serious it is and how basic a change in brain chemistry must cause it. The pattern of Margaret's sleep loss is typical of the illness. Psychiatrists use the term *early morning awakening* to refer to this particular sleep disturbance. Patients report that they fall asleep more or less quickly and at the normal time but wake up very early in the morning, often at two or three o'clock. They often say this is the worst time of the day, a time when they, as Margaret put it so succinctly, "obsess about every foolish thing I've ever done in my life." The mood often lifts as the day goes on. This pattern of mood change throughout the day, worst in the early morning hours and improving throughout

the day, called a *diurnal variation in mood*, is a classic symptom
of the depression seen in affective disorder. *Diurnal* comes from
a Latin word meaning "of the day."

"Has there ever been another time in your life when you had
these kinds of problems?" I asked.

"Not that I can remember."

"How about after the birth of your children? Did you notice
any depression then?

"Well, now that you mention it, I did have crying spells for
about two months after David was born. I'd just burst into tears
for no reason. But isn't that normal? I think my mother called it
'the baby blues.' She said it would pass, and it did."

Here was another piece of information that is strong evidence
Margaret was suffering from the depression of affective disorder—
a prior episode. This is another of the hallmarks of affective disorder: its episodic pattern and tendency to recur. As is frequently the
case, Margaret's first episode was milder and shorter than the one
that brought her to medical attention. As is also too often the case,
it went unrecognized and in fact was explained away as being
"normal."

Other diseases were once thought to be normal, especially very
common ones. For example, many people, including many physicians, believed "getting senile" was a normal part of growing old.
We now realize that a specific disease process causes the insidious
loss of memory and other types of intellectual deterioration sometimes seen in elderly persons. This condition, like Parkinson's disease, is now thought to be caused by the death of cells in a particular
brain center, the nucleus solitaris. This illness is the now-familiar
Alzheimer's disease, more properly called Alzheimer's type dementia.
It was named after the physician (who was a psychiatrist, by the
way) who first described it. This "senility" is a disease process, and
there is nothing normal about it.

Similarly, symptoms of affective disorder at particular times
of life have been called normal or explained away as a psychological

reaction to certain life events. "The baby blues" is one example. We now know that hormonal changes can be associated with changes in mood and that postpartum depression (*postpartum* being the medical term for the period immediately after giving birth) probably has a significant chemical component. It doesn't happen to everyone, and how well or poorly one adjusts to motherhood does not predict who will get it.

The most striking example of how affective disorder has been misunderstood in this way is the story of "involutional melancholia." For many years it had been noticed that severe depression sometimes occurs in women going through menopause. Like postpartum depression, it was often explained in psychological terms. In this case it was seen as a psychological reaction to the termination of reproductive life—a kind of mourning for the end of the childbearing years and the beginning of old age. What was ignored was that the symptoms did not look at all like mourning but had all the characteristics of the depression of affective disorder. When effective medication for depression became available, it was found to work for involutional melancholia. It seem illogical to call an episode of the depression of affective disorder by another name when it happened to occur at menopause, so the name was dropped as a diagnostic category. (I'll be returning to these issues in a later section called "Mood Disorders in Women.")

"How has this change in mood affected your working, your free time?" I asked Margaret. "What do you do for enjoyment?"

"Usually I can really relax and enjoy myself after dinner with my painting. It's always been such a source of pleasure for me. But I don't enjoy it as much as I used to. I just can't get interested in it. I'm exhausted by the end of the day."

"Would you say you don't get as much enjoyment out of a lot of things anymore?"

"Well yes, I suppose that's true. I just sort of feel stuck; I can't do anything to pull myself out of it. David's team won their first soccer game of the season this past Saturday. Last year I got so tickled watching them, even if they lost. Now every game is a chore. I get so restless and irritated at the thought of spending an afternoon at the school. God, I lost my temper on the way home last week just because the poor little kid had gotten grass stains on his uniform. I've been a real bitch to live with."

Another classic symptom: *anhedonia*. The word is derived from a Greek root meaning "pleasure" (a hedonist is someone who lives only for pleasure). Anhedonia is inability to experience pleasure. Again, it is by discovering the qualities of mood change that are abnormal that a psychiatrist make the diagnosis of affective disorder. Sad persons who are not suffering from affective disorder usually do not have marked anhedonia. Usually they are able to shake off their sadness for a time during the day and enjoy some pleasurable activity. They can go to a movie and forget their troubles for a few hours or take a drive in the country and come back refreshed. A person in the midst of the depression of affective disorder, however, cannot escape from a continuous, pervasive change in mood that is simply unrelenting. The mood is consistently the same—miserable. Some little pleasure or happy accident during the day that ordinarily would cheer the sufferer just falls flat. Remember I said earlier that normal mood is reactive. In affective disorder the mood loses this quality—there is no reaction to events in the environment. This phenomenon has been called a *constriction* of mood.

"I want to shift gears a bit and ask you some questions about your family background," I said. "Do you know if anyone else in your family—parents, brothers and sisters, anyone at all—has ever needed to see a psychiatrist or take medication for depression or emotional problems?"

"No, nothing like that."

I persisted. "Now I want you to think carefully about your mother and father, aunts and uncles on your mother's side." Margaret's face became a little more strained in concentration. "Aunts and uncles on your father's side."

"My uncle Edgar, on my father's side, was in a mental hospital once . . . no, I think it was two or three times."

"What can you remember about your uncle?"

"Well, it's funny, because he always seemed perfectly normal to me. They raised five children who all turned out just fine. Come to think of it, I never could make sense out of what my mother said about him."

"How so?"

"Well, she told me he had had shock treatments in the hospital. I thought you really had to be crazy to need that. But as I said, he always seemed just fine to me. He owns a big dry-cleaning chain in the West; he works hard, makes tons of money. He sure seems happy and healthy now."

Well, I thought, this pretty much ties it up: a family history of a psychiatric problem severe enough to require hospitalization that was treated with electroconvulsive therapy. There were a number of questions to be asked for the sake of completeness. But Margaret's family history, her own history, and her symptoms made quite a case for a diagnosis of the depression of affective disorder.

The Symptoms of Major Depression

Let me review the process that led from Margaret's family doctor's description of her as "depressed" to a diagnosis of affective disorder. First, and most important, Margaret reports feeling depressed. She does indeed feel a change in her mood as I described mood in the first chapter. Important also is that she can date the onset of the change and clearly states that she feels very different now than she does when she is her usual self. Interestingly, some patients with the depression of affective disorder say they do not feel particularly depressed. Usually they seem to mean they are not sad and do not feel like crying, but they certainly are unhappy. They seem to be simply miserable, very irritable and short-tempered, impatient and restless, unable to relax, unable to say anything nice about anything or anybody.

Secondly, Margaret reports that her mood change is with her every day. It is pervasive, there all the time, interfering with everything she does or wants to do. Many patients find that the mood change even intrudes on their sleep in the form of unpleasant dreams. Themes of death, loss, and pain are frequent. Abraham Lincoln, who undoubtedly suffered from affective disorder, had dreams of death and dying during the depressions that haunted him episodically for years. Shortly before his assassination, he told his wife he had dreamed of finding a corpse lying in state on a catafalque in the East Room of the White House. Whether this was some kind of mystical revelation of his own impending death I will leave to the parapsychologists, but it was certainly a typical symptom of the depression of affective disorder.

Margaret's depressed mood has some qualities that are seen in affective disorder and are not usually seen, or at least are not very prominent, in other types of depression. These qualities are her feelings of guilt and failure and her anhedonia. This loss of interest in usually pleasurable activities is very important. It seems to grow out of the pervasiveness of the mood change. As I said earlier, psychiatrists sometimes call this a constriction of mood or, as I have described it, a loss of the normal reactivity of mood.

Margaret has been preoccupied with some thoughts and issues that did not bother her before she got depressed, specifically her adequacy as a mother. Many patients with depression find that their minds continually return to the same unpleasant thoughts. Even though they try to put such thoughts out of their minds, their mental activity is drawn to the same depressing theme as if by some force like magnetism or gravity. In psychiatry such ideas are called obsessional thoughts or simply obsessions. Many people who are not depressed have similar experiences—we have all heard some melody, maybe something silly like an advertising jingle, and found ourselves humming or just thinking it throughout the day; even though we try to push it out of our minds, it keeps coming back. An obsessional thought is similar but usually is unpleasant and is resisted by the patient, who tries to think about other things, but without success. Several years ago I treated a depressed man, a devout Catholic, who was tormented by recurring thoughts of having sexual intercourse with the Virgin Mary. Not only were these thoughts extremely distressing in themselves to this religious man, but such blasphemous and therefore "sinful" ideas compounded the feelings of guilt caused by his depression. Another patient had the recurrent fearful thought that she was going to accidently start a fire, so she began to avoid matches and soon even the stove in her own kitchen. Patients with obsessional thoughts cannot push them away for long and sometimes will complain of the fear of "losing my mind" to express their alarm at these out-of-control experiences. When obsessional thoughts are symptoms of affective disorder (and many are), they disappear when the disorder is properly treated.

Another common experience is the feeling that one's thought processes are slowed and inefficient. One may believe one's memory is bad, since when we aren't concentrating well it is hard to remember things. This slowing and inefficiency are also responsible for the indecisiveness depressed people often feel. This symptom seems especially prominent in older persons who become depressed (see "Major Depression in the Elderly" in chapter 5). Sometimes people who are severely depressed take longer to think and speak, and even their movements can be slowed down, an effect called *psychomotor retardation*. (*Retardation* here has its literal meaning of "slowed" and has nothing to do with the term *mental retardation*, which refers to low IQ.) This lethargy is sometimes interpreted as laziness by those around the sufferer, and their criticism can compound the guilt associated with the illness.

Margaret is having vegetative symptoms of depression; that is, she notices changes in her usual bodily activities and rhythms. She has noticed a change in her appetite and a change in her sleeping habits. There is a particular pattern in her sleep disturbance, too: early-morning awakening. Some people have sleep and appetite changes in the opposite directions when they are depressed; they find that they sleep and eat more than is usual for them.

The uncomfortable physical sensations accompanying the depression of affective disorder can at times be so distressing that they dominate the clinical picture. Many people simply feel "sick" or "tired" in a vague and general way, but others notice a variety of true pains. Headaches are very common, as is a sense of heaviness in the chest. Any little ache that might otherwise be ignored seems to be exaggerated and becomes more difficult to endure, so that back pains or arthritis pains seem much worse (see "Pain and Depression" in chapter 5). Constipation is another common complaint.

Margaret reports a loss of interest in sex. This symptom may be thought of as an aspect of anhedonia as well and is very typical of the depression of affective disorder.

These symptoms point to affective disorder, but other information Margaret supplied was also helpful in making the diagnosis.

She gave a history of prior unexplained mood change (her "baby blues") that lasted several months and went away spontaneously. Affective disorder follows what physicians refer to as a relapsing and remitting course. It is episodic in that there are relapses separated by long periods of remission during which there are no symptoms. More about this aspect of the illness later.

Last, she told me that a blood relative had had a psychiatric illness severe enough to require hospitalization but had recovered completely. Another important piece of information is that he received electroconvulsive therapy. We'll discuss this much maligned but safe and effective treatment later. For now I'll just say that it is now used almost exclusively for severe episodes of the depres-

Table 1   Common Symptoms of Major Depression

Depressed Mood

    Pervasive, constricted quality of depression
    Feelings of guilt and inadequacy
    Fearful, overwhelmed feelings
    Onset of a fear of being alone
    Diurnal variation in mood
    Preoccupation with failure, illness, or other unpleasant themes
      (may become obsessional thoughts)
    Nightmares, especially with themes of loss, pain, or death
    Anhedonia (loss of ability to experience pleasure)
    Indecision
    Onset of unexplained anxiety, panic attacks

Vegetative Signs

    Sleep disturbance (too much or too little, especially with early
      morning awakening)
    Appetite disturbance (increased or decreased, usually enough
      to cause weight change)
    Fatigue, low energy
    Vague aches and pains, heaviness in the chest
    Constipation
    Loss of interest in sex
    Poor concentration, slowed thinking, (psychomotor retardation)

sion of affective disorder. The genetic (hereditary) link in affective disorder is very strong. As we will see later, having a relative with affective disorder greatly increases one's chances of having the disorder (see "Heredity of Mood Disorder" in chapter 6).

Psychiatrists now have pretty much agreed on a term for the depression of affective disorder. Margaret would be diagnosed as suffering a *major depressive episode*, and her illness—her type of mood disorder—is called *major depression* (see table 1).

Other Types of Depression

In discussing Margaret's symptoms, I used the phrase "other types of depression." In the very first section I posed the question, What is normal mood? and answered that a good or happy mood is not the only normal mood. (As you will see later, a good mood can be abnormal too.) Now that we have talked about abnormal depression, the mood disorder called major depression, a reasonable question to consider is: Can there really be such a thing as "normal depression"? Let's examine this question by considering another case:

Patty is a seventeen-year-old high-school student who came to my office with her mother. Mom did most of the talking:

"Doctor, we're so concerned about our Patty; her father and I are very worried that she's depressed." Patty's mother was a pert, animated woman who wanted the best for her family and impressed me as a "take charge" type of person who was going to get it.

"What kinds of things make you worry that she is depressed?"

"Well, she just looks so gloomy and sad all the time. She mopes around the house; she doesn't go out with her friends like she used to. She's not as interested in school as she was. She's just not the old Patty."

Patty had always been a good student; in fact, she still was. She seemed to do less homework and to be less concerned with school, but her marks were still at about the same level as they had always been. Patty agreed that she didn't feel like going out with her friends the way she had during the previous school year and over the summer. She admitted that school wasn't as interest-

ing as last year, and she had to force herself to do the bare minimum of homework to maintain her grades.

Her mother mentioned that Patty had broken up with a boy-
friend recently, but Patty, rolling her eyes with an "Oh, Mom" look,
corrected her and said that the breakup had occurred months ago
and she was over it. Patty had done a little experimenting with
alcohol and marijuana, but I believed her when she said she had
tried them only a few times.

Her mother told me that Patty's older brother had had a
severe bout of depression but was doing much better now that he
was taking medication. This piece of information was a red flag,
and as I continued to question Patty and her mother I felt the
evidence was compelling for a diagnosis of major depression. I am
going to discuss the treatment of affective disorder at length, so
I won't go into the details of Patty's treatment with medication
now. But I felt there was enough evidence of a mood disorder for
a therapeutic trial and prescribed some medicine. Besides the
family history, she had a change in mood that seemed not to be in
response to anything, not understandable in light of her recent life
events. After starting her on medication, I saw Patty weekly to
assess how her symptoms were responding and as I always try to
do, I tried to get to know her better, constantly refining the diagnosis and treatment plan. As sometimes happens, when I found
out more about her my formulation of Patty's problem changed.

Patty's best friend was Audrey, and they did everything together. The new school year had started several months before,
and for reasons they couldn't quite understand, there was a
change in the pattern of friends they shared. Patty and Audrey
suddenly found themselves part of the "popular crowd" at school.
Patty had always been popular, but she considered herself a bit
shy. Now she got invited to the best parties, ate lunch with the
"popular crowd" in the cafeteria, and so forth. A teenage girl's
dream come true, isn't it? Well, Patty certainly felt that way at
first, but she started to change her mind as the school year went
on. She found her new friends flashy but shallow. The "best"
parties turned out not to be as much fun as last year's parties
with her old friends, and Patty thought there was too much drinking. Her family was Baptist and strongly discouraged any use of
alcohol; although Patty was not as rigid as her parents, teenagers

getting drunk definitely bothered her. She found a lot of the girls catty and cruel and the boys "stuck-up" and sexually aggressive.

Audrey, on the other hand, thought their newfound clique was *the* group to be with and couldn't understand why Patty had become so "uncool." Patty found herself in a real dilemma; she felt uncomfortable with her new friends and their values but felt she couldn't go back to her old friends or get different new ones without losing Audrey's friendship. (Remember that Patty thought of herself as shy.) Mom and Dad were rather strict parents, so Patty felt she couldn't really discuss these things with them (especially the "sex and booze" part).

Patty missed the "good old days" of last year. On the other hand, she was a senior and was really looking forward to college. She was confident that her marks were good enough to get her into the school she wanted, but she wondered if "college kids" were going to be like the new group she was feeling uncomfortable with. What if she didn't fit in any better at college than she did now? She felt a little trapped in the current situation and had some worries about the future. As adolescents often do, Patty had a very hard time seeing her current loneliness and feelings of alienation as temporary and situation limited.

Of course it took several sessions for me, a stranger, to get all of this out of an adolescent. During those weeks, as I was gathering all this information, it was becoming clear that the medication wasn't having much effect. One week Patty told me she had spent a couple of days at her grandmother's house in the country and had run out of her pills. Not only did she not feel worse without them, she actually felt better than she had in a while. It turned out she usually had a wonderful time at her grandmother's farm. It was like a return to the carefree days of childhood, and she felt refreshed by the change in atmosphere and time away from her social pressures. I told Patty to stop the medication, but I kept seeing her every week to talk about the problems at school. We talked about how to handle peer pressure, how friends sometimes grow apart as they grow up, about "shyness" and self-confidence. Her mood got better and better with psychotherapy and without medicine.

The question this case leads me back to is, Can depression be normal? Let's examine what I said about a normal mood change. I described it as understandable and proportional. In Patty's case it took a while for me to figure it out, but when I did her mood change indeed had these qualities. Patty's nostalgia for past relationships, feelings of not fitting in, fears of losing her best friend, and so on make her changes in behavior, such as not going out with friends as much and losing interest in school, understandable. Also, although she worried that she was shy (and this was not new, according to her mother), Patty did not have the preoccupation with inadequacies or guilty feelings that is typical of major depression.

As we shall see, mild cases of affective disorder sometimes lack many of the typical symptoms, but given Patty's continued improvement even after her medication was stopped, one is hard pressed to say she suffers from an illness.

Nevertheless, one is also reluctant to say this behavior is normal. If by "normal" one means "the way it should be," clearly teenagers shouldn't be depressed. On the other hand, considering Patty's story and thinking about what we know of the emotional reactions people usually have to conflicts, our intuition and our own experiences inform us why Patty's mood and behavior have changed. We do not have to invoke a disease process disrupting normal functioning to explain these changes. On the contrary, knowing Patty well and considering the situation that developed in her environment, we might almost predict some of her uncomfortable feelings as the expected result.

Yet, Patty definitely had a problem in the emotional realm that was uncomfortable, impaired her to some extent, and required and responded to treatment, albeit psychological treatment, not medication. What was my diagnosis of Patty's problem? In the latest version of the classification of psychiatric problems of the American Psychiatric Association, Patty would be said to be suffering from an adjustment disorder with depressed mood. The key features of this diagnosis are that there is an identifiable stressor (the stress in this case is the social change and disruption of relationships that have occurred) and that there is some impairment of functioning. In Patty's case the impairment was not severe, it would be little more than her decreased socialization with her peer group and her "moping" around the house. Although not listed in the formal classification of psychiatric disorders, the term *reactive depression* is still often used to discuss this type of mood change. It is still a useful concept and brings me to another important topic.

The Classification of Depression

As you have seen from reading about Margaret and Patty, the phrase "I'm depressed" can describe what almost seems to be two different conditions. Margaret clearly has an illness, Patty seems to be reacting in an understandable way to life circumstances—yet they are both depressed. Their problems appear similar and yet, intuitively, they seem different. Even before neurochemical evidence accumulated for a biological basis for some changes in mood, psychiatrists recognized these types of differences and wondered if there were different kinds of depression. When medical treatments for depression were developed it was discovered that not all who complained of depression could benefit from the new treatments. This led to attempts to differentiate the types of depression that did benefit from those that didn't and some new clinical terminology was developed.

In older textbooks of psychiatry one reads various clinical terms that attempt to classify depression, usually, into two basic types. *Primary* depression, as opposed to *secondary* depression, refers to depression that seems to arise "out of the blue" rather than being caused by a life event and thus secondary to or following on something else. *Endogenous* and *reactive* depression express much the same meaning. The word *endogenous* is from Greek roots meaning produced or growing from within; *reactive* is used with its customary meaning indicating that something is a result of an external event. These terms still are used quite frequently, but as we shall see, there are some problems with them.

Psychotic depression and *neurotic* depression are expressions that have largely fallen into disuse, and for good reason. A psychosis is a condition characterized by loss of contact with reality and is certainly an imprecise term at best. While some cases of the depression of affective disorder are severe enough to cause "psychotic" symptoms, such as hallucinations, the vast majority are not. Neurosis has meant little more than "every emotional disorder that isn't a psychosis." After several attempts to define neurosis more precisely, psychiatry has largely abandoned the term.

Another way in which these differences have beeen expressed is to speak of "depression the symptom" and "depression the syndrome." A symptom is basically a complaint made by a patient. Chest pain, shortness of breath, and ringing in the ears are all symptoms. Depression is a symptom, too, and like the other symptoms I mentioned it may indicate one of several underlying problems but is not seen exclusively in any one. A syndrome, by contrast, is a whole collection of symptoms and other findings that point strongly to a particular diagnosis or small set of diagnoses. Pain in the wrist, for example, accompanied by swelling, redness, and heat constitutes the inflammatory syndrome, or more simply inflammation. To specify that the inflammation is in a joint, we use the term *arthritis* (from Greek *arthron*, "joint"). The pain is the symptom: the swelling and so forth that the doctor notices on examination are called "signs." The syndrome is arthritis, and there are limited causes for this syndrome.

The depressive syndrome includes the symptom (complaint) of depression (or more precisely, depressed mood), but it also includes many other symptoms: anhedonia, the quality of guilt and self-reproach, as well as other signs that go beyond the mood alone: vegetative signs, diurnal variation of mood and so forth. Taken all together, these symptoms and signs define the *depressive syndrome*. Everyone has experienced depression the symptom, but only people with affective disorder have the syndrome of depression. (Actually, some other causes of the syndrome are possible, as you'll see in chapter 6 under "Medical Causes of Mood Disorders" and elsewhere.)

Why all this interest in classification? Perhaps instead of *classification* I'll substitute a more familiar word that doctors use: *diagnosis*. Diagnostic categories are really systems of classifying diseases. The basic organizing principle in a system of diagnostic catagories is prediction of treatment and outcome. Making a particular diagnosis allows the doctor to predict which treatment will be most effective in getting the patient better. The obvious advantage of accurate diagnostic classifications is that the most effective treatment can be chosen quickly, eliminating unnecessary treatment by ineffectual methods.

In the treatment of depression, several facts have been discovered that make diagnosis important: the medications and other treatments I will be discussing in the next chapter provide the most benefit in cases of endogenous or primary depression: the syndrome of depression. Persons with reactive or secondary depression often do not derive any benefit from these sort of treatments but instead get better with a very different kind of treatment: psychotherapy. Conversely, patients with features of endogenous depression cannot usually get better with psychotherapy alone; medical treatment is necessary. Although the endogenous/reactive dichotomy seems the best system to address the issue of predicting treatment response, it is not perfect. The depression of affective disorder can follow a traumatic event and seem reactive, yet respond to medication. In addition, some forms of psychotherapy can be very useful in the treatment of persons who have depression with endogenous features.

Let's examine another case history in order to understand these issues more clearly:

Robert is a thirty-six-year-old engineer who has just been through a nasty divorce from his wife of ten years. They have three daughters aged nine, eight, and two. Robert and Nancy had not been a very compatible couple from the start and began to have difficulties early in their marriage. Robert was a serious, methodical, rather meticulous person who wanted a quiet home-life, while Nancy was a vivacious, independent, at times tempest-uous woman who was impulsive and could be almost reckless in her pursuit of new experiences. In the early years of their relation-ship the temperamental differences between them were comple-mentary and mutually enriching. Robert and Nancy were the opposites that attract. As the years passed, however, these differ-ences caused more and more problems. The large age gap between their older daughters and their youngest occurred because Nancy decided (several years after she and Robert had agreed they would have no more children) that she also wanted a son. Without informing her husband, Nancy stopped taking her birth-control pills. When she became pregnant she thought it was a great joke on her serious-minded husband. Robert, however, interpreted Nancy's actions as complete disregard for his feelings about their family's future. Sexual intimacy between them practically stopped because Robert felt he could not trust Nancy not to get pregnant again. They began to bicker and grow distant. Robert spent more and more time at the office. One day he came home to find Nancy and the children gone. He discovered that Nancy had left him and taken the children to her hometown three hundred miles away.

A long and acrimonious divorce process began. Unfortunately, Nancy's volatile nature and need for confrontation made every disagreement on terms a battle of wills. Every issue was a source of bitter contention and custody of the children was the most emotional and nastiest battle of all. The arrangement that eventually was painfully worked out was joint custody, Robert having the children with him each summer and during the week between Christmas and New Year.

Despite a legal document clearly outlining each one's rights and responsibilities, and even with several hundred miles separating them, Nancy and Robert continued to have disagreements that precipitated violent verbal confrontations. In many ways Nancy missed Robert very much, but her pathological independence made it impossible for her to compromise to solve their problems. The thought of Robert leading a life of his own seemed to enrage Nancy, and she used every interaction with him to act out her fury in the most petty ways. Robert would travel three hundred miles to pick up the children at an agreed time only to find Nancy's house empty. She would return hours later with the children and simply say she had been grocery shopping. Robert would get abusive phone calls in the middle of the night accusing him of not sending his support payment; he would investigate the matter at the bank and stop payment on the check, then Nancy would tell him the check had mysteriously appeared in the mailbox.

Throughout his trial by fire, Robert maintained his usual steady and methodical manner in his work, went through the wrenching process of selling the house their family had been growing in, and simultaneously met Nancy's assaults on his peace of mind with what could only be described as equanimity. His unflinching even-temperedness prevailed as Nancy's histrionic energy waned, and their relationship settled into an uneasy truce, or at least a cease-fire.

Six months after the divorce, Robert still found himself preoccupied by the devastation wreaked in his life. Instead of beginning to put the event in perspective and getting on with rebuilding his life, however, Robert ruminated on the past and tortured himself with questions. Had he been too hard on his wife? Had he been too rigid and unyielding? What had he done to change her high spirits and zest for living into bitter, recriminating sarcasm and conflict?

Robert found it difficult to concentrate on his work. He lost weight. His colleagues commented that he looked tired all the time. He wondered if he had some kind of infection and went to see his family doctor.

"I heard about Nancy the other day, Bob," the doctor said as he walked into the examination room. "I'm sorry things got so bad between the two of you. Listen, I'm sure she'll be back to her old self in a few weeks."

"I don't know what you're talking about."

The doctor looked somewhat pained and very embarrassed. "Oh, God, you mean no one's told you what she did?"

"No. What?"

"Nancy took an overdose two days ago. The hospital they took her to called me for her medical records. Fortunately her medical condition wasn't too serious. I think they were going to admit her to the psychiatric unit."

You're probably wondering at this point, Who's the patient here? Well Robert was my patient, Nancy was somebody else's. Clearly they were both very unhappy people and both suffered from depression. Whose depression was more severe? The answer is obvious or so it would seem. Nancy became so distraught that she decided life wasn't worth living and tried to kill herself, didn't she? Robert had a bad mood that went on for a while, but he was a "neurotic," introverted guy anyway, wasn't he? Isn't his depression understandable?

The treatments that eventually resulted in both their recoveries were very different. Robert took antidepressant medication and got better. Nancy was admitted to the hospital, her doctor did *not* start her on an antidepressant (as Robert reported later). Yet she also got better. Let's consider the cases one at a time, try to classify their depressions as endogenous or reactive, and examine the treatment each doctor chose.

Robert's mood problem did not really begin until after most of the conflict with Nancy had ended. I described Robert as a logical, methodical person who did not like surprises or discord. If anything would "drive him crazy," that is, cause him to have severe reactive symptoms, it would have been all the conflict during the time immediately following their separation and divorce. One would expect him to begin to feel better once the dust had settled. When we look at the quality of his depression, we identify symptoms of guilt and self-recrimination. Robert also had persistent and marked appetite and sleep disturbances. His history is strikingly like Margaret's. Robert's depression is major depression: he is having a major depressive episode.

How does the fact that he had a severe emotional trauma fit into the clinical picture? It was once emphasized in psychiatry that when a precipitating event could be identified, the diagnosis of major depression was unlikely. This has clearly not turned out to be so. Instead, we now recognize that emotional trauma can precipitate an episode of affective disorder—the death of a loved one, the loss of one job, or as in this case, a divorce.

A metaphor I often use to explain this concept to my patients is the common experience of getting caught in a soaking rain, becoming chilled, and then coming down with a cold. We know that getting chilled doesn't *cause* colds; viruses cause colds. But the chill can cause a set of biological circumstances that allows a virus in the air to get a "foothold" in the upper respiratory tract and bring on a cold. It may be that emotional trauma causes a similar set of circumstances that allows an episode of affective disorder to occur at that particular time in a vulnerable person.

Physical stress can also precipitate an episode of affective disorder, especially certain kinds of physical stresses. The physical stresses in women associated with childbirth, menstruation and menopause as well perhaps as some specific hormonal changes during these times can cause the depression of affective disorder. (I will discuss this further in the chapter on variations of affective disorder.)

It is because the depression of affective disorder can follow on an emotional or physical stress that the term *reactive depression* should be used cautiously. The term *adjustment disorder* (Patty's diagnosis) is now used in the diagnostic manual of the American Psychiatric Association to denote the relation between precipitating event and subsequent depression.

■ ■

Now what about Nancy? The first step in her psychotherapy will be to get to know her better—her growing-up years, her family, her personal assets and vulnerabilities, the ways of coping with adversity that she used to deal with her problems over the years. This is what Nancy's therapist learned about her in the first several weeks of her therapy:

As you remember, Nancy is in some respects Robert's opposite; where he likes predictability and routine, Nancy thrives on the new and unexpected. One of Nancy's problems, which can be understood as an aspect of these qualities, is that she is impulsive. Robert tends to approach a problem logically and carefully—he will consider options, weigh pros and cons, then make a well-reasoned decision. Nancy, on the other hand, will listen to her feelings and intuition and decide issues almost spontaneously, often based on emotion rather than logic. She will pick a particular option because it "feels right."

Another problem is that Nancy reacts very badly to loss and rejection. She had had a difficult childhood, to a large extent because her parents died in a car accident when she was two years old. Nancy was shuttled between several different sets of relatives as she was growing up, raised by various aunts and uncles who considered her a burden and an intruder into their own families. As a child Nancy never knew when she would be uprooted and sent on to yet another family. After a few years she started to act up whenever she sensed that her guardians were getting tired of her. Rather than face yet another rejection, she would reject first. She was not conscious of this pattern, but it was almost as if she reasoned on some unconscious level, "You don't think I'm good enough for your family; well, I'll show you what bad really is!" In an unfortunate and destructive way, Nancy protected her fragile self-esteem by giving her aunts and uncles good reason to get rid of her. This led to an even more difficult tendency; it became extremely hard for her to admit when she was wrong. She blamed others for her own lapses of judgment and her impulsive and foolish decisions: "If you hadn't treated me that way, I wouldn't have done it." The idea of admitting she had been wrong and asking forgiveness as a prelude to working out differences was anthema to Nancy.

How does this added knowledge about Nancy help us understand the problems between her and Robert and even more important, her suicide attempt? Her impulsiveness may explain the "unplanned pregnancy" that seemed to set off the unfortunate chain of events culminating in divorce. Then when Robert rejected her sexually, Nancy, sensing that he might want to end the marriage reacted (impulsively) by leaving him. As she had often done before, she blamed Robert completely for their problems; she remained furious at him, and her anger poisoned his attempts to placate her or reason with her. The custody and child-support battle became an emotional battering ram that Nancy could not resist using against him. Yet, in her moments alone, Nancy missed Robert and yearned for the happy early years of their marriage.

Now that we have some more background let's look more closely at Nancy's depression and her suicide attempt. In addition to her reaction to the interpersonal loss, Nancy did not like being a single parent. Finances were tighter, so she had to work part-time. This left little time or energy, let alone money, for a social life. This "all work and no play" was very difficult for Nancy. Robert, who had always found work stimulating and even soothing, could throw himself into it and gain a therapeutic effect. For Nancy work was something one did to get money for fun, and given her financial situation she wasn't getting much fun for her efforts.

As she might have expected, her relatives were less than supportive of her, either emotionally or financially. "So you've screwed up again" was the reproach she could detect behind their cool politeness as she visited her aunts and uncles in the old hometown. Their thinly veiled sarcasm was more than she could stand, and she stopped her contacts with them. As the months passed Nancy became more and more unhappy. She felt trapped in a situation not of her own making, abandoned once again by those she had been foolish enough to trust. She became increasingly angry, lonely and depressed. One day she dropped the children off at school, went home, and took an overdose of sleeping pills. She then tried calling Robert to let him know what he had done to her, but couldn't reach him. She began to panic and dialed 911 before she lost consciousness.

Now that we have gotten to know more about Nancy it becomes apparent that her problems are very different from Robert's in many respects. Nancy has a set of attitudes about herself and others that make life difficult for her. Because of some destructive childhood experiences, she reacts in maladaptive ways to certain kinds of problems, especially problems in her relationships. Often her reactions, even the well-intentioned ones, make things worse rather than better. Understanding Nancy's particular personality vulnerabilities and considering the events leading up to her overdose one does not need to invoke a disease process disrupting normal functioning and imposing itself to understand her mood change and actions. Nancy's feelings and actions almost seem normal—for Nancy. Well, *normal* is of course not the right word, better to say they are understandable in the light of her personality traits and the unfortunate set of circumstances to which she is reacting. And there's that word—*reactive*.

Clearly, giving Nancy medication to restore the balance of neurotransmitters is off the mark. Her problems are much more complicated, deeper really, and grow out of her personality and approach to life. Her treatment will consist of helping her to put aside her anger at Robert, giving her support and encouragement in addressing the immediate problems in her life, and over the longer term helping her understand how some of her feelings and reactions to problems are rooted in the past rather than appropriate to the present. Clearly this is in the realm of the psychological rather than biological.

If classifying and diagnosing depression is so tricky, you might wonder, why not treat everyone who complains of depression with medical treatment and psychotherapy both? Many studies actually indicate that a combination of both is most effective. Nevertheless, medications and other medical treatments have side effects and risks and psychotherapy can be a long, often very expensive process and also has associated risks. When bankrobber Willie Sutton was asked why he robbed banks, he replied, "Because that's where the money is!" In the treatment of depression both physician and patient want to put their efforts "where the money is" when making treatment decisions. Although there are certainly many cases of depression that fall into the grey zone, there are many that are clearly black and white and where emphasis on medical *or* psychological treatment needs to predominate.

These case histories also illustrate a problem with the term *major depression*. Robert has major depression, yet Nancy almost killed herself. *Major depression* seems to me to imply something catastrophic or at least extremely severe and it is in many ways an unfortunate term. The word *major* may be taken to mean that the depression of affective disorder is always incapacitating or florid in its symptomatology. In reality, some people never have symptoms severe enough to bring them to medical attention of any kind, much less psychiatric treatment. They simply go on in misery, perhaps thinking that everyone feels as bad as they do but that they can't cover it up as well as others. Many people with this disorder have a smoldering debilitating problem that goes on for years and years, like an ulcerated sore that does not heal. They become so accustomed to their chronic misery that they just learn to live with it.

There is another set of terms that describe this smoldering, chronic type of depression: *dysthymia* and *dysthymic disorder*. The prefix *dys-* in medicine denotes abnormal or impaired, and the root *thymia* refers to the mood. Dysthymic disorder is a diagnosis in the latest edition of the official classification of psychiatric disorders used by the American Psychiatric Association, the *Diagnostic and Statistical Manual of Mental Disorders*, third edition, revised (the DSM-III-R). It refers to a mood disorder that is not as severe as a major depressive episode but goes on for a long time. To meet the diagnostic criteria for dysthymic disorder, the patient must be symptomatic with a depressed mood most of the time for at least two years. Other diagnostic criteria are similar to those used to describe major depression—appetite and sleep disturbance, low energy, low self-esteem, and so on. Simply put, *dysthymia* refers to depression that is chronic and smoldering but not florid or terribly debilitating.

One can imagine that a person with the depression of affective disorder can have symptoms of depression that are not as severe as major depression for two years and thus meet criteria for dysthymia. But one can also imagine that somewhat maladjusted individuals who are in chronically difficult relationships or who hate their jobs but can't or won't leave them or have other severe ongoing problems might also fit the picture. So is dysthymia a reactive or an endogenous depression?

Earlier in this section I mentioned all the terms that psychiatrists have used to try to classify depression, *endogenous depression, reactive depression, primary, secondary, neurotic, psychotic*. I've already mentioned *major depression* and now *dysthymia*. Why all these terms? The existence of so many classification systems for depression illustrates a simple fact: psychiatry has not yet come up with diagnostic categories that accurately separate those cases of depression that will respond quickly to medication from those which will not. In fact, the DSM-III-R does not even address treatment in its system of classification lest it get caught up in the ongoing debates about the causes of various forms of depression. Instead, the manual concentrates on describing clinical syndromes without discussing underlying diseases, sources of symptoms or treatment issues. For the sake of simplicity, I will continue to use the term *depression of affective disorder* to refer to depression that seems rooted in abnormal chemistry of the brain and which requires medical treatment.

If this discussion of the classification of depression seems confusing to you, it's confusing to clinicians also, so don't be discouraged. There are some simple facts, however, upon which almost every expert agrees: although not all persons who are depressed will derive benefit from medical treatments for depression, some persons who have depression suffer from an illness rooted in the biological or chemical functioning of the brain. Medical interventions are necessary in the treatment of these patients and psychological treatment alone will usually not be very effective.

THREE

TREATMENT

The Treatment of Major Depression

Now that we have discussed the symptoms of major depression it is time to turn to its treatment. As I said in the first chapter, a large body of evidence has accumulated to indicate that mood disorders have as their basis a change in the chemistry of the brain. When a person develops the combination of symptoms of depression I described in the last chapter, it seems that they are caused by a change in the balance of neurotransmitter activity in the brain. It makes sense then to approach this problem with medical treatments that somehow affect the chemistry of the brain.

Medications

As has often happened in medicine, drugs used to treat mood disorders were discovered practically by accident. Effective medications were found and successfully used for years before scientists had a clue to how they worked. In fact, there has been a sort of reverse investigation in understanding the chemistry of depression and the chemical effect of these medications. The discovery of how they change brain chemistry has pointed the way toward a biochemical theory of affective disorder.

Antidepressants

One of the most revolutionary developments in treating emotional problems with medication was the discovery in the 1940s of chlorpromazine (Thorazine). This drug was found to alleviate many of the symptoms of a very different illness from the one that concerns us here—the devastating chronic psychiatric illness schizophrenia. Chlorpromazine treats the hallucinations and disrupted thought processes of this disease in a very specific way.

Medications had been used in treating schizophrenia for many years, but they were really little more than "knockout drops" that put patients to sleep or sedated them. The development of chlorpromazine made available for the first time a drug that did not simply quiet an agitated person but seemed to relieve the symptoms of the illness without affecting other brain functions such as level of consciousness.

Professor Roland Kuhn of Zurich reasoned that if a medication could control the symptoms of schizophrenia in this specific way, there must also be a chemical way to treat abnormal mood states. He literally pulled some drugs off the shelf and tried them on depressed patients. (Actually, he tried a number of drugs that had originally been synthesized as possible antihistamines but were abandoned when their activity proved weak.) He became convinced that one of them, at first known only as "G22355," had an effect on the abnormal mood states of his depressed patients. In 1958 he published a paper in the *American Journal of Psychiatry* called "The Treatment of Depressive States with G22355 (*Imipramine Hydrochloride*)." The first antidepressant had been discovered: imipramine.

The first generation of antidepressants are all chemically similar to this original one. Their names bear this out: amitriptyline, nortriptyline, desipramine. Another one that is also chemically similar is doxepin. A drawing of the chemical structure of these drugs would show that they all have three connected rings of atoms. For this reason they are often referred to as tricyclic antidepressants.

In the years since the introduction of the original antidepressants, more have been developed. Some of their names are trazodone, amoxapine, and maprotiline. These drugs, sometimes referred to as second-generation antidepressants, are useful because they have a different profile of side effects (see table 2).

What do these drugs do? For many years, because the chemical activity of the brain was so mysterious, the mechanism by which antidepressants work was completely unknown. More recently, study of the effects of these drugs in the brains of animals and sophisticated chemical brain-mapping techniques have revealed various effects on brain chemistry, but their mechanism is still far from clear. One problem is that different antidepressants that are equally effective in treating affective disorder may differ considerably in their effects on the brain. For example, amitriptyline considerably boosts levels of the neurotransmitter serotonin and to a lesser extent norepinephrine. Another and usually equally effective medication, nortriptyline, has a similar effect but in an opposite pattern, boosting norepinephrine more than serotonin.

At one time researchers thought there might be two kinds of depression in affective disorder, one characterized by a relative deficiency of the neurotransmitter norepinephrine and another caused by a relative deficiency of serotonin. Much work has been done on by-products of these chemicals that can be measured in

Table 2   Common Antidepressants and Their Brand Names

Tricyclic Antidepressants

     Amitriptyline (Elavil, Endep)
     Nortriptyline (Aventyl, Pamelor)
     Protriptyline (Vivactil)
     Desipramine (Norpramin, Pertofran)
     Doxepin (Adapin, Sinequan)
     Imipramine (Tofranil, Imavate)

"Second-Generation" Antidepressants

     Amoxapine (Asendin)
     Fluoxetine (Prozac)
     Maprotiline (Ludiomil)
     Trazodone (Desyrel)

MAO Inhibitors

     Tranylcypromine (Parnate)
     Phenelzine (Nardil)

the spinal fluid. It was thought that by measuring the levels of these by-products one might differentiate between the theorized types of biological depression. Although some are still convinced that this line of research will eventually be very fruitful, the results of most of these studies have been equivocal at best and therefore unconvincing to most neuroscientists. (This is the "MHPG" literature you may come across in older books and articles; see "Tests for Affective Disorder" later in this chapter.) Whether one antidepressant or another is better in treating major depression is a matter of controversy. Studies of large groups of patients have never shown that any of the available antidepressants is superior in effectiveness. Attempts to classify biological depression chemically have not been successful, and no single theory of brain chemistry explaining the effects of antidepressants has emerged. It may be that their chemical effects in the brain that we can measure bring about a more basic biological change we cannot measure, and that it is this more basic effect that treats depression.

So, unfortunately, I can't say much about how antidepressants work except that they change the chemical activity in the brain. I do want to tell you about the experience of taking antidepressants and what a course of antidepressant therapy is like.

One of the biggest problems with antidepressant medications is that they take a comparatively long time to bring about their effect on symptoms. Unlike aspirin, decongestants, antihistamines, antacids, or other medications you are probably familiar with, the therapeutic effects of antidepressants are not apparent in a few minutes or hours. In fact, their effects usually become apparent only after weeks—roughly, two to four weeks. It is not entirely clear why this should be. That this time lag is unexplained should of course not be surprising, since the basic mechanism by which antidepressants work is largely unknown. Some facts about brain chemistry that are known, however, do provide some possible explanations.

First, the nerve cells and their chemistry are separated from the chemistry of the rest of the body by the *blood-brain barrier*. Some substances penetrate this barrier very slowly and therefore take much longer to have an effect. Since a medication taken by mouth must be absorbed into the bloodstream and then pass the blood-brain barrier, some delay may occur at this step.

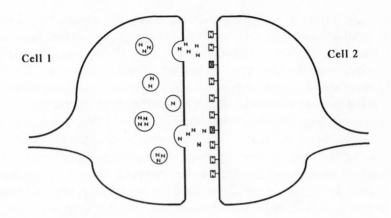

Figure 2   How neurotransmitters activate nerve cells.

ɴ = Neurotransmitter   ◻⊦ = Receptor
▨⊦ = Neurotransmitter-receptor complex

Also, various substances have very gradual effects on brain
chemistry because they cause a change not in neurotransmitters
but in the receptors on the nerve cells. Remember that the neurotransmitters are chemicals that flow across a tiny space from
one nerve cell to another to carry their "on/off" message. (The space
is called the *synaptic cleft*.) When they get to the other side of this
space they switch the next cell on because they fit into a receptor
on the surface of the cell as a key fits into a lock. There are many,
many receptors, and a critical majority of them must get the on
message for the next cell to fire. Let's look at this process more
closely (see fig. 2).

To understand some things about neurotransmitters and their
receptors, let me compare some of their properties with a more
familiar example of information carriers: You probably have in your
wallet or purse a bank card or credit card that you can use to get
money out of an automatic bank teller machine. For you to get money
on a particular day, several things must occur. First of all, of course,
you must have sufficient funds in your account. I'll assume you're
a frugal person who always does. Now two other conditions are
necessary: you must have your bank card with you, and you must
find an automatic teller machine for your bank. There must be a
match between type of card and type of machine for you to get

money. When the match is correct, the transaction takes place.

Now imagine that in your town there has been a rash of robberies of people using their cards to get cash and that suddenly nobody wants to use the machines. Since fewer people use the machines and they are expensive to maintain, your bank starts removing them. As weeks go by it becomes more difficult to complete your transaction because there are fewer machines and therefore there is less opportunity to make a correct match.

Let's imagine that a year or so goes by and memory of the robberies fades; also, many new people move into town who want automatic teller service and ask for bank cards. There are a lot of cards in town now, so the bank responds by increasing the number of machines. After the several weeks it takes to install them, it's easy once again to complete your transaction.

What has this to do with brain chemistry? Think of a neurotransmitter as the bank card and the receptor as the slot of the automatic teller machine. When the neurotransmitter flows across the space between cells, there are receptors on the other side. The neurotransmitter must match a receptor for the message to be transmitted just as the right kind of card must get into the slot of the right kind of teller machine. The number of "transactions" depends on the number of receptors as well as on the amount of neurotransmitter. Neuroscientists are discovering that nerve cells can regulate the number of receptors on their surface in response to the amount of neurotransmitter activity. Just as the bank changed the number of teller machines in town based on its customers' card use, a nerve cell can increase or decrease the number of receptors on its surface based on the amount of neurotransmitter activity. And just as it takes time for the bank to recognize the change in demand for its machines, hire the contractors to remove or install machines, and get them ready for business, brain cells also have a "turnover time" for receptor changes.

I told you earlier that understanding the effects of antidepressants on the levels of neurotransmitters in the brain has not led to a coherent theory of the biology of affective disorder. I said it may be that the chemical effects we can measure bring about a more basic biological change we cannot measure, and that it is this more basic effect that treats depression. Well, there is compelling evidence that the more basic biological change has to do with receptors. Neuroscientists are discovering that in many cases the turnover time for neurotransmitter receptors is—you guessed it— two to four weeks, the same time it takes antidepressants to work. It may be that antidepressants take several weeks to work because of the time needed for receptor changes to occur.

Getting back to symptom response, not only does improvement take weeks, it also has a peculiar pattern described by Dr. Kuhn in the first patients to take antidepressants. He noted that his patients' families often saw improvement before the patients themselves did. This has been consistently observed with all types of antidepressants.

Here is a typical story: A man notices that a week after she starts on antidepressants his depressed wife is taking more interest in her appearance, and he points out that her medication must be beginning to work. "Are you kidding? This stuff isn't doing anything for me," she says. "I still feel terrible." But a week later she has to admit her mood is better.

Often an improvement in sleep is the first sign. The patient falls asleep more easily and sleeps through until morning. No more "early morning awakening." The appetite is better and weight loss stops. I can usually tell when antidepressant medication is working in my patients at least a week before they themselves notice any improvement. Sometimes the change is almost too subtle to put into words—a slightly more erect posture, a smile here and there during our appointment.

In my office I have several options for where my patients can sit. I always sit at my desk. The patient can sit facing me in a regular office chair beside my desk, or on a small, rather low sofa against one of the walls, also facing me but a little farther away. I never tell my patients where to sit; if they ask I tell them to sit "wherever you like." Again and again I have seen the following pattern: when patients come to see me who are very depressed, they first sit on the sofa almost slumped over and sinking into the cushions. After taking antidepressants for several weeks they sit closer, taller, more energetically in the office chair. Even if they don't report feeling much better, this change tells me we're on the right track.

Notice that I have been using the term *treat* rather than *cure*. There are some diseases that medicine can cure. Penicillin can kill all the bacteria causing pneumonia, and that's the end of the disease. It's cured. It won't come back again unless a new infection occurs.

What about high blood pressure, though? There are medications that will lower high blood pressure to normal levels, but as soon as the patient stops taking them, the blood pressure rises again. The problem is treated with the medication, but the underlying disease process is not reversed. In many cases the symptoms will return if the treatment is not continued. The treatment of affective disorder is much like the treatment of high blood pressure. (As a matter of fact, some of the same chemicals are involved. Remember reserpine?) Antidepressants seem to treat the symptoms, but if the medication is stopped they can come right back.

Notice I said they *can* come right back. Back in chapter 2 I said that affective disorder follows a relapsing and remitting course, meaning that the symptoms will eventually go away by themselves. Thus psychiatrists often talk about an *episode* of affective disorder. In this disease the episodes of relapse can be separated by long periods, many years in most cases. Whatever the change in brain biology that occurs when the symptoms of affective disorder come on, it eventually reverses itself and the symptoms go away. This means that the patient must continue to take medication during the entire time that the episode lasts. This turns out to be between six and eighteen months *on average*. As we shall see later, some other forms of affective disorder have a very different course, and the length of time on the medication is highly variable.

What about side effects? The good news is that there are practically no really dangerous side effects. Some of the older antidepressants can cause certain problems with the rhythm and organization of the heartbeat in people with certain kinds of heart problems. But there are very few people who cannot take them for this reason.

The bad news is that there are a lot of annoying side effects of many of the antidepressants (see table 3). Fortunately, these usually diminish with time. The side effects of the traditional antidepressants tend to be worst during the first few days of treatment, and they are usually minimized by starting the medication at a low dosage. This means that a patient may start taking a dose of antidepressant that is only one-quarter or even less of the amount needed to get the full benefit of the medication. For example, most patients need 100 to 150 milligrams of imipramine to get complete symptom relief, but most get intolerable side effects if they start out at more than 25 or 50 milligrams a day. I usually raise the dose every third or fourth day to begin with, then increase it more slowly as the dosage gets higher.

As you can see by counting the days it takes to get from a starting dose to a full dose and then adding on the time needed for the full dose to have its effect, it will sometimes be *three to five weeks* before there is significant improvement. Some newer antidepressants (fluoxetine is one) work at low doses, and there is generally no need to gradually raise the dose; but even these still take two to four weeks to have an effect.

Many patients of mine report feeling "spacy" or "out of touch" during the first few days on antidepressants. These symptoms usually pass, but they may crop up temporarily each time the dosage is increased. Some of the antidepressants are sedating—that is, they promote sleep. These are of course very useful in persons who are

Table 3　Common Antidepressants and Some of Their Side Effects

Medication (Generic Name)	Anti-cholinergic Effects[a]	Sedation	Weight Gain	Other
Amitriptyline	3+	3+	2+	
Desipramine	2+	—[b]	——	
Doxepin	2+	3+	2+	
Fluoxetine	——	——	——	Nausea initially; possible weight loss
Imipramine	2+	1+	——	
Maprotiline	1+	2+	2+	
Nortriptyline[c]	2+	1+	——	
Trazodone	——	3+	——	Painful penile erections (rare)
Phenelzine	——	1+	1+	Special diet;[d] insomnia, dizziness
Tranylcypromine	——	——	——	Special diet;[d] insomnia, dizziness

[a]See text for complete description of these side effects.
[b]Almost none.
[c]Very accurate blood-level test available.
[d]See text on MAOs.

having sleep problems. Others are somewhat stimulating and for this reason cause sleep problems. Again, this may be useful in patients who find themselves lethargic and sleeping too much. But some patients will find this stimulation unpleasant and complain that the medication makes them jumpy and anxious and interferes with their sleep.

Some antidepressants promote weight gain because they increase appetite; again, these may be useful in people who have lost weight because of depression. A more recent antidepressant has been shown to be something of an appetite suppressant in some patients.

Antidepressants can cause episodes of dizziness, really an exaggeration of the common experience of feeling lightheaded when getting up suddenly from sitting or lying down. Most patients report that this gets better after a few days, and most cope with it simply by taking their time standing up, being especially careful to get out of bed slowly in the morning when blood pressure is low anyway, and sitting on the edge of the bed a few moments before standing up.

Most of the tricyclic antidepressants partially block the neurotransmitter acetylcholine, which is instrumental in some of the automatic functions of the body, including the activity of the digestive system and the focusing of the eyes. One of the results of this blockade is dryness of the mouth caused by the suppression of the salivary gland function. Some people experience constipation as well. The focusing problem makes it difficult to read fine print. These are called anticholinergic side effects. They usually get better in time, but I tell my patients they may need to chew sugarless gum to stimulate the flow of saliva and use a bulk laxative for a week or so. (If patients stop taking an antidepressant with anticholinergic activity too quickly, the gastrointestinal tract seems to "speed up" again, and some people have mild, temporary nausea or diarrhea.)

The anticholinergic side effects can cause a variety of urinary problems too. In some people they interfere with the nerve impulses necessary for emptying the bladder. This is usually a problem only in older men, at the age when the prostate gland (absent in women) surrounding the duct that empties the bladder can enlarge and narrow the opening. A man who has trouble emptying his bladder after starting on an antidepressant needs to stop the medication and call his doctor.

There is a difference between a side effect and an allergy to a drug. An allergy is an abnormal immune reaction to something new to the body. It is caused by the response of the body's immune cells to the new chemical and usually takes the form of a skin rash or fever; in rare cases there are blood-cell problems, and in even rarer cases, the catastrophic anaphylactic reaction in which the blood pressure suddenly drops, the bronchial tubes (the breathing passages to the lungs) swell shut, and cardiac arrest can occur. Remember that a person can be allergic to just about anything, and who is allergic to what is simply impossible to predict. People who are truly allergic to a medication *cannot* continue to take it. Since antidepressants are synthetic compounds and most allergies are to naturally occurring substances, usually proteins, true allergies to these medications are fortunately rare.

Side effects, however, are common; almost every drug has some. Some unwanted effects of medication often go along with the wanted effects and cannot be separated out. When you take a shower, you can't get clean without getting wet; it's impossible to separate one effect from the other! Fortunately, the desired effect (cleanliness) lasts longer than the side effect (wetness), and the side effect is tolerable, by most at least. So it is with medication side effects. It is important to remember that side effects do not mean one must stop taking a drug, only that one is faced with a choice: Is the therapeutic effect of a particular medication worth putting up with the side effects? Sometimes another choice is available, and sometimes the side effect is treatable. For example, a mild laxative will usually clear up the constipation caused by some antidepressants.

As I stated earlier, the antidepressants all seem equally effective in treating major depression. Some people have better results (better *antidepressant* results, not just fewer side effects) from one than from another, though, so if one antidepressant doesn't work there may be some benefit in switching to another. The choice of which one to prescribe, however, is largely determined by the side effects, and not all antidepressants cause the same profile of side effects. For example, some of the newer ones have almost no anticholinergic side effects, but many of them are very sedating. One of the frustrating problems for patient and doctor is that it is impossible to tell which side effects a particular patient will have, or at least which will be so bad that another antidepressant must be tried. There is often some trial and error involved in antidepressant therapy.

The point I want to make is that antidepressant treatment is not something to be either entered into or abandoned impulsively. Unlike, say, a cold preparation, the medication will not show its benefits for weeks, and in the meantime the side effects many be somewhat uncomfortable. Another point is that since there are many antidepressants, with different side effect profiles, it is important that the patient tell the doctor if intolerable side effects develop so that a switch can be made as soon as possible.

I find that the second or third week of antidepressant therapy is the most difficult for my patients. This is the time when they are having the most side effects and seem to be getting little if any benefit. This is when patients are prone to what I call the "flush reflex." This is the tendency to give up on medication and—you can guess the rest.

Some of the most frequent reasons for the "failure" of antidepressants are inadequate prescribed dosage, not taking the full dose, and not persevering long enough for the medicine to work.

In the past several years, reliable laboratory tests have become available to test the amount of some antidepressant medications that actually gets into the bloodstream at a given dose. It has been discovered that people vary tremendously in the way their bodies handle antidepressants. Some need much higher doses than others to get the same level in the bloodstream. This may account for why people vary in the dose they need to get a full antidepressant effect from a particular drug. For many of the antidepressants, it has been determined just what the blood concentration of a drug should be for the patient to receive the optimal therapeutic effect. These tests are useful in the patient who is taking what is usually a reasonable does of antidepressant (100–200 milligrams a day for most [not all!] drugs) but does not seem to be getting any better. If the blood level is low, a higher than usual dose may be necessary (and safe). If the level is therapeutic, it indicates that a different medication or another type of treatment may be necessary.

Another bit of good news is that more and better antidepressants are constantly being developed. The antidepressant fluoxetine (Prozac) became available between the time I started writing this book and the final revision; there will undoubtedly be more types available by the time you read this.

A last point about antidepressants: their only effect is to reverse the symptoms of major depression. They are not "happy pills"! For many people, the only drugs they know that affect mood are drugs of abuse. From what they have read or perhaps even experienced, they know that certain drugs induce in just about everyone who takes them a feeling of euphoria known as a "high" or "rush." The term *mind altering* or *mood altering* is sometimes used to describe this effect. Because drugs like cocaine, heroin, and amphetamines, to name a few, have this effect in everyone, they are liable to be used solely for the sake of this effect. In some people the pursuit of the high becomes compulsive until it is the dominant activity in their lives, often to the exclusion of family life, school or work, and so forth. Seeking out the drug's effect begins to take up more and more of their energy, and they may even engage in crime. An additional quality of some drugs that produce a high is that the body becomes habituated so that larger and larger doses are required to produce the same effect. Neuroscientists and psychiatrists sometimes argue about the meaning of the word *addicting* and about which drugs are physically as opposed to psychologically addicting. "The pursuit of the high" seems like a pretty good working definition of what addiction is.

Antidepressants do not produce euphoria. A person taking an antidepressant who does not suffer from major depression will experience no change in mood whatever. Thus these drugs are not abused; any drug dealer foolish enough to sell imipramine would soon be out of customers! They are not on the list of "controlled substances," medications prone to abuse, of the Federal Drug Administration.

The body does not become habituated to antidepressants. Some patients confuse the procedure of raising the dose with the need addicts have to take more and more of their drug of abuse to get their high. With the antidepressants, once the proper dose is reached, no further increases are necessary, nor does the patient have any desire to increase the dose.

Antidepressants are not addicting by any criterion or definition. They are not "mind altering" or "mood altering" either. Patients sometimes fear that the medication will somehow change them or alter their personality. "I don't like the idea of taking something that's going to work on my brain!" is a comment I often hear. I think of antidepressants, and all the medications and treatments used in mood disorders, as "mind restoring" or "mood restoring." They don't really change anything except the symptoms of affective disorder. They take away the abnormal feelings, thoughts, and physical symptoms that are caused by the illness and return patients to their normal state.

Other Medications Useful in Depression
MAO INHIBITORS

There is another class of medications, chemically quite different from the more commonly used antidepressants, whose discovery and use in the treatment of depression was almost simultaneous with that of imipramine. This class is related to drugs originally developed to treat tuberculosis, and they interested psychiatrists when one of them was noted to alleviate depression in some patients taking it for tuberculosis.

More investigation revealed that this class of medications could increase the levels of nervous system amines (the chemical class of many neurotransmitters). Since the observation had been made a few years earlier that reserpine depleted amines, it was theorized that this new class of drugs might help in depression. Clinical trials confirmed an antidepressant effect.

These drugs take their name from their action on the enzyme monoamine oxidase (MAO). An enzyme is a substance that causes a particular biochemical action in the body, and MAO is responsible for deactivating various amines, including neurotransmitters. MAO-inhibitor medications essentially deactivate this deactivator, thereby increasing the level of amines.

Why does the body have the enzyme MAO in the first place? Because various amines are constantly entering the bloodstream. Epinephrine, also known by the more familiar name adrenaline, is one. When stress or a frightening event occurs, the adrenal glands pour out adrenaline, causing the heart rate to increase, pupils to dilate, blood pressure to rise, and so forth. The body needs a way to turn off these reactions when the fright is over. This is where MAO comes in; it essentially gobbles up the adrenaline, terminating the effects.

A large amount of MAO is found in the lining of the intestines. This is because some breakdown products of digested proteins resemble adrenaline closely enough that they would cause an "adrenaline rush" if a lot were absorbed quickly and not immediately deactivated by MAO.

Patients taking an MAO inhibitor must adopt some special precautions, since this medication blocks one of the body's defenses against adrenalinelike substances. These substances crop up in the most surprising ways. Any food that contains large amounts of the amino acid tyramine must be avoided, and this turns out to include all kinds of goodies like certain cheeses, wine, and beer. Many cold medications contain drugs that have the same effect. If patients taking an MAO inhibitor ingest a food or medicine that contains one of these chemicals, it affects them like a shot of adrenalin. The most serious problem is the rise in blood pressure that ensues, which can be so severe that it causes a "hypertensive crisis." Such a sudden rise can rupture blood vessels in the retina of the eye or even in the brain. Symptoms of stroke and even deaths have been reported, although this is extremely rare.

Because of these problems the MAO inhibitors were quickly eclipsed in use by their cousin imipramine and its "descendants," the rest of the tricyclics and other medications described above. MAO inhibitors caught on a bit more in England, where they are even today often the first type of antidepressant prescribed. In the United States they are becoming more popular as doctors become less afraid to use them. They really are quite safe if a few precautions are taken. Nevertheless, they are usually reserved for patients who do not respond to the other classes of antidepressants, and they sometimes produce a dramatic response when a traditional antidepressant has been ineffective. Less frequently, an MAO inhibitor is added to a traditional antidepressant and the two are taken together.

THYROID MEDICATION AND OTHER HORMONES

When I discuss tests for depression I will be mentioning that various thyroid hormones are being investigated for their utility in diagnosing depression. The thyroid hormones, which set the rate at which the body uses energy and "burns" calories, seem to be affected in mood disorders, especially major depression. Sometimes they also play a role in its treatment. A depressed patient whose thyroid gland is the slightest bit underactive will respond poorly to antidepressants. In some depressed people, even if the thyroid hormone level seems normal, adding a small dose of thyroid medication seems to boost the effect of the antidepressants and turn an incomplete response into a complete remission of symptoms.

In women small doses of estrogen, the main "female" hormone, sometimes have the same effect.

LITHIUM

Another drug that is often very helpful in treating major depression is lithium. I will postpone a full discussion of this medication until the chapter on bipolar disorder (manic-depressive disorder), since lithium is much more frequently used for this variation of affective disorder; nevertheless, interest is growing in its antidepressant uses. Here I'll say only that switching to lithium or adding it to an antidepressant sometimes increases relief from depressive symptoms.

STIMULANTS

Stimulant medications similar to the amphetamines, now used in children to treat attention deficit disorder (hyperactivity), were at one time used extensively to treat depression. They fell out of favor because they are so prone to be abused (as "uppers" or "speed") and because clinical trials looking at their efficacy as a sole treatment for depression were unconvincing. Recently there has been renewed interest in their use in combination with traditional antidepressants. The most commonly used stimulant is methylphenidate (Ritalin). Their use in major depression is still highly controversial.

TRANQUILIZING MEDICATIONS

As you will see further on, the symptoms of depression can become extremely severe; the sleeplessness can be completely exhausting, and sometimes the patient can be overwhelmed with distress and even agitation. I've mentioned that one of the problems with antidepressant medications is that they take quite a while to work. Fortunately, there are other medications that can make the depressed person a bit more comfortable until they do.

Although in mild cases the usual medications for anxiety and sleeplessness (the *sedative/hypnotics*, hypnotic referring to sleep, not hypnosis!) are effective in relieving these symptoms, patients with major depression often get better relief with the stronger tranquilizing medications that were first used (and are still used) to treat schizophrenia. These medications have been called by several names, including *major* tranquilizers (as opposed to *minor* tranquilizers, which are used for mild anxiety and insomnia), neuroleptics, and most commonly now, antipsychotic medications. The first antipsychotic was chlorpromazine (Thorazine), and another one that is commonly used in major depression is thioridazine (Mellaril). I've already talked about the problems with the word *psychotic*. Although the term is a pretty good one when one considers the fact that the primary use of this class of medications is in schizophrenia, the term *antipsychotic* shares the same impreciseness and bad connotations of its parent word. Nevertheless, this term is usually used in discussing this class of medications and so I will use it as well.

In major depression the antipsychotics are used as tranquilizers: that is, they are used to reduce anxiety and tension and promote sleep. Also, some patients become so profoundly depressed as to lose touch with reality (as we will see in the case of Sylvia in the next section) and antipsychotics may have a specific effect on some of these very distressing symptoms. Although they are often very helpful for these problems, they do not by any means take away all the symptoms of depression. For example, they have little effect on the low mood. Nevertheless, they can considerably reduce the overall distress of the very depressed person while other treatments are beginning to work.

Before more widespread use and experience with antidepressant medications, antipsychotic medications, and especially thioridazine were thought to have some antidepressant effects of their own. This idea has been for the most part abandoned, although some think antipsychotics may help the antidepressants work better in some patients.

An important point to remember is that these medications are symptomatic treatments. This means they are used to help some of the symptoms of the illness such as sleeplessness and anxiety while the underlying mood disorder is more slowly resolved through the effects of the antidepressant or other treatment. As you'll see later, antipsychotic medications are even more useful (and also often more necessary) as symptomatic treatments for another clinical form of affective disorder, the manic state. Once the underlying mood problem has been controlled, however, the symptomatic treatment is no longer necessary, and there is hardly ever any reason for a patient with affective disorder to take this type of medication long term.

As with any other tranquilizers, the most common problem with the antipsychotic medications is oversedation. If the dose is too high, the patient may feel sleepy, groggy, or "drugged." The simple solution is of course merely to lower the dosage.

The antipsychotics seem to work by blocking the neurotransmitter dopamine. As you may remember from chapter 1, this is the neurotransmitter that is low in Parkinson's disease. Therefore, as you might expect, a medication that blocks the effect of dopamine can cause the same symptoms—stiffness, shuffling walk, tremor, and so forth. Indeed, some of these symptoms do occur sometimes in patients taking antipsychotics. Other movement problems can also occur, including muscle spasms, especially of the head and neck. As with oversedation, these side effects usually get better if the dose is lowered. If a patient cannot tolerate a lower dosage because of the severity of depressive symptoms, the drugs used in Parkinson's disease are very effective in treating these side effects; in fact, some psychiatrists almost automatically prescribe an anti-Parkinsonism medication at the same time as they prescribe an antipsychotic.

In patients who take antipsychotics at high doses for many years, a movement disorder called *tardive dyskinesia* can develop. This problem takes the form of continual small muscle movements, usually affecting the facial muscles. Patients with this problem seem to always be making chewing movements, pursing their lips, or wrinkling their noses. There is no medication to reverse tardive dyskinesia, but usually it gradually goes away if the antipsychotic is stopped. For patients with mood disorders, use of antipsychotic medications is usually so brief (days or perhaps weeks) that the problem almost never develops.

I hesitate to spend too much time on the side effects of the antipsychotics, since they tend to sound much more terrible than they really are. They can be uncomfortable until treated, but they are certainly not dangerous. These medications are almost always a temporary measure, and just as a narcotic pain medication provides temporary relief of physical pain, they provide valuable and usually welcome relief of the terrible psychic pain of severe depression. Like narcotics, they are strong drugs whose use is to be taken seriously and monitored closely. (By the way, unlike narcotics, the antipsychotics are NOT addicting, habit forming, or liable to be abused.)

There is a pharmaceutical preparation, very frequently prescribed at one time, that combines amitriptyline (an antidepressant) and perphenazine (an antipsychotic) in the same pill. A preparation that combines two or more medications in this way is called a "fixed combination." Although some patients certainly do take both an antidepressant and an antipsychotic for a time, almost none need to continue the antipsychotic for long, and so the short-term usefulness of such a combination seems to me to be outweighed by the inability to vary the dose of the components independently.

It may seem I am belaboring the point about symptomatic treatment. But all too often, symptomatic treatment of mood disorders has taken the place of definitive treatment of the underlying problem. Before the use of antidepressants became widespread and more doctors became skilled in their use, it was not uncommon for a person who complained of some of the symptoms of major depression to simply be given sleeping pills or sedatives. One reason the fixed-combination preparation I mentioned above was so widely prescribed was that it had "a little of this and a little of that" (a little antidepressant and a little tranquilizer) and was almost guaranteed to make things a little better no matter what the problem! Usually, however, if the problem was major depression, although some of the symptoms got a little better, the patient was still depressed because there wasn't enough of the antidepressant. Especially in mild cases, this bit of symptom relief might be sufficient to persuade depressed persons that it wasn't necessary to see a psychiatrist after all, and so they would suffer for many more months until the depression went into remission on its own.

Electroconvulsive Therapy

Perhaps no treatment in medicine has been so unfairly maligned as electroconvulsive therapy (ECT). Several years ago a jurisdiction in California went so far as to outlaw its administration. Fortunately, soon after this foolish law was passed the facts about ECT were presented to the electorate and the law was repealed. More than fifty years after its introduction, after remarkable refinements in technique and, most important, after incontrovertible proof of its safety and extreme efficacy, there are still well-educated and sophisticated people who say they would never allow it to be given to themselves or their families.

As has so often happened in medicine, a series of coincidences led to the discovery that an electrical treatment could alleviate severe depression. The key word here is "severe": I will give some examples of the kind of depressions that require ECT in the next section. Suffice it to say here that only about two-thirds of severe depressions respond to medication, yet over 90 percent respond to ECT. I've always thought the best way to learn about a treatment is to understand its history, so let me review the history of ECT.

At the turn of the century, someone observed that people with epilepsy—those who had episodic uncontrolled spasms of electrical brain activity taking the form of convulsions or epileptic seizures—seemed to have a lower incidence of mental illness. This observation turned out to be an error; as a matter of fact a number of distressing emotional symptoms are often seen in those with some forms of epilepsy. Nevertheless, this led to the study of seizure activity in humans in search of a treatment of emotional symptoms. Experiments were performed in dogs to determine if a method could be developed to cause seizures without serious side effects. After work with various drugs and inhaled substances, it was determined that a seizure could be induced relatively safely by passing a small electrical current through the skull from electrodes applied to the scalp. In 1938 two Italian psychiatrists reported their success in treating depressed patients with this technique.

After a number of years and initial resistance, the treatment became widespread, for a very good reason: it was a seemingly miraculous "cure" for an illness that until then had no treatment. (Remember, the first antidepressants were developed in the 1950s.) Patients who had been so depressed that they were literally starving from lack of eating or had been suicidal for months were completely free of their symptoms of depression in a matter of days. The reasons for the recovery were completely unknown, but it was clear that this amazing treatment could produce astonishing improvement in some patients.

But ECT's success was also its downfall. It was so effective in some patients that it was overprescribed and used in others with very different psychiatric problems, for whom it offered little hope. Even this is to some extent understandable, however, since in the early part of this century there were no medications to treat any form of emotional disorder. The severely mentally ill often were simply locked up in institutions for months and even years with no hope of returning to normal. Could one deny such a person a trial of any treatment that had even the slimmest chance of helping? Unfortunately, however, ECT seemed to be labeled a treatment of last resort for hopeless cases.

Another problem was that there were some complications. An epileptic seizure can be a violent event. Patients suffered broken bones, wild fluctuations in blood pressure, and even abnormal heart rhythms that could lead to death. These problems added up to a very bad reputation for ECT, a reputation exploited by some in the entertainment industry, who portrayed ECT in movies as a sadistic, bizarre torture method used by evil psychiatrists to punish troublemakers (*One Flew over the Cuckoo's Nest* comes to mind).

Fortunately, there were courageous doctors who were unwilling to give up a proven therapy because of the ignorant hysterics of a few strident extremists. They continued to refine the technique, and as anesthetic methods improved, the incidence of problems associated with the treatment dropped dramatically.

Today ECT is administered in an operating room or a special treatment suite in hospitals. Using safe anesthetic techniques, patients are put into a deep sleep just as if they were to undergo surgery. One of the anesthetics used completely relaxes all the muscles, so that the actual "seizure" is an electrical event only. No jumping or jerking occurs in a properly anesthetized patient. On the contrary, the patient remains practically motionless, and only some minor changes in pulse rate and blood pressure indicate that anything at all has happened during the one second or so that the tiny electrical current passes through the skull. The entire treatment lasts ten to fifteen minutes.

How does this treatment work? This remains one of the most

deeply shrouded mysteries in psychiatry. We know that the therapeutic effect of the treatment is directly related to the seizure activity. Simply passing a current through the skull is not sufficient; seizures must be induced. Why a seizure should have an effect on mood evokes little more than vague speculation among neuroscientists. Because the chemistry of mood is so poorly understood, and because the effect of seizure activity is so difficult to measure, there are only a few guesses even today. The levels of various neurotransmitters are elevated after ECT, but as with the antidepressants, so many neurotransmitters are affected that no particular pattern has been implicated as either cause or cure. Some have pursued lines of thought suggested by the therapeutic effect of electricity in correcting abnormal heart rhythms.

For years electrical current has been passed through the chest in patients whose hearts are not beating correctly. (The use of resuscitation paddles is familiar to even the most casual television medical show fan.) Like the nervous system, heart muscle cells conduct tiny amounts of electricity. As this tiny current reaches each cell, the cell contracts. For the heart to pump properly, the current must pass through the cells in a smooth, organized pattern. Think for a moment of a team of rowers. They must all pull in unison for the boat to move forward. If they all were to row in their own rhythms, chaos would result and the boat would not move in any direction but would simply flounder about. When the heart becomes diseased or injured, as when there is a sudden blockage in one of its blood vessels, its electrical activity can become disorganized and the cells can begin to contract out of rhythm. The most severe form of this asynchrony of contraction is fibrillation. A heart that is fibrillating does not pump; each cell is contracting in its own rhythm, and the heart simply quivers. By passing a current through the heart (the machine used to deliver the current is called a defibrillator) the cells are shocked into contracting simultaneously. In this way they are synchronized again and contract in an organized fashion so that the heart once again beats and pumps.

Back in chapter 1, I mentioned that the brain system that regulates mood may not be concentrated in a small area of the brain but may constitute a network of nervous fibers spreading out through many areas. Some have suggested that in affective disorder such a system is discharging its electrical and chemical signals in an abnormal rhythm and that ECT sets its functioning right much as the defibrillator corrects the heart rhythm. This line of reasoning is logical and rather elegant, but it is strictly theoretical speculation at this point.

Unlike defibrillation, however, ECT does not produce its effect after a single treatment. Usually eight to twelve treatments are necessary, so psychiatrists usually speak of a *course* of ECT. One treatment is given about every other day in most hospitals. Usually this is done on a Monday, Wednesday, Friday schedule. Therefore a course of eight to ten treatments means a hospital stay of three or four weeks. Usually, by the fourth or fifth treatment improvement in mood is noticed by others and perhaps even reported by the patient. Often there is a peculiar temporary recovery in mood immediately, even after the first treatment. For several hours the patient will have a striking improvement in mood state, but as the hours pass depression sets in again. With each treatment this improvement lasts longer and longer, and eventually it is sustained from one treatment to the next. Soon the patient feels completely back to normal.

How is the length of a course of treatment determined? Once I was invited to a dinner party given by some friends who had worked in Morocco in the Peace Corps. Each guest was to bring an authentic Moroccan dish. Since most people don't have Moroccan cookbooks at home, the hosts kindly provided them. The book I got was, well, primitive in its directions. Besides its calling for ingredients like pigeon, the cooking instructions were very vague. My favorite one, which ended nearly every recipe in the book, was "cook until done." No oven temperature, no length of time in the oven, just "cook until done."

The answer to when to stop giving ECT is not much more exact. "Stop when the patient is better." I've heard advice to give treatments until the patient is completely recovered, then give one more! This is of course something of a simplification. If after several weeks of treatment there has been no response, the diagnosis of depression must be questioned and other diagnostic evaluations and treatment methods investigated. Eight to twelve treatments is an average.

Another note on the efficacy of ECT. Whereas the depression of affective disorder usually lasts several months and an antidepressant must be continued for the entire period, ECT not only treats the symptoms but also seems to terminate whatever internal process causes the mood change in the first place. Once recovery is complete, that episode seems to be ended in many people, and no further treatment is necessary. Nevertheless, many psychiatrists start their patients on antidepressants after successful ECT just to make sure the symptoms don't come back. Whether this is really necessary remains somewhat controversial.

What are the side effects of ECT? As you might suspect, the major side effects of the treatment come from the anesthesia, not from ECT itself. Patients awaken from anesthesia a bit groggy and confused for a time. Most of this confusion wears off almost immediately, but in some patients it may last an hour or two. This seems to happen especially in older people and also those who have had brain injury from one cause or another, such as a stroke or an auto accident. In these persons the disorientation can last much longer. When this happens the treatments can be given less frequently over a longer period. Confusion that lasts more than a few hours is worrisome, however, and may indicate that the patient is suffering another problem in addition to depression that requires evaluation. Serious episodes of confusion usually mean that the treatment course should be reconsidered.

The best known—or rather the most notorious—side effects of ECT concern memory. Although memory problems have been reported for many years, their types and extent have been evaluated in an organized way only over the past ten years or so. It was at one time suggested that the memory loss was the reason ECT worked—that people "forgot their problems" after receiving it! This was soon proved false, since no correlation was found between therapeutic effect and extent of memory loss. The problem of memory is still controversial because it has been difficult to measure some of the types of memory loss patients report.

Most experts agree that ECT seems to interfere with the consolidation of memory for the time when the patient is receiving the treatments as well as for a short period before and after. This means that memories for events that occurred during the three weeks or so that a typical patient is in the hospital getting ECT may be foggy or even completely lost forever. In addition, some memory for events in the weeks leading up to the hospitalization may be lost. This is called retrograde amnesia, *retro-* meaning "back" and in this case referring to the period before the course of ECT.

In addition to this pattern, patients sometimes report that they temporarily lose memory for isolated events that occurred years before the ECT or lose other bits of memory in an almost random fashion. I heard of a patient who needed to look up a favorite recipe that she had made without a cookbook for years. It's almost as if a tiny snippet of memory has been clipped out for some people. Usually, however, these memories too return with time. As you might imagine, it has been very difficult to devise tests to confirm such memory losses.

Although many patients report no memory problems whatever, and most have only minor and temporary difficulty, some people do report feeling that their memory has never been the same.* I'll only comment that these complaints seem rare in my patients, most of whom are very thankful that a treatment is available that alleviates their symptoms so quickly.

Are there patients who cannot be given ECT? Yes, those who are serious anesthesia risks—patients with certain severe heart problems or respiratory disease. But other than these very ill people, there are few; patients with brain tumors, for example, are usually excluded. ECT can be given to persons who have recovered from heart attacks, to persons with epilepsy, and with careful monitoring and skilled anesthesia, even to pregnant women. Old age is not a barrier; in fact, there is considerable evidence that ECT is especially effective in the elderly and perhaps safer than some of the antidepressants (see "Major Depression in the Elderly" in chapter 5).

Complicated Depression

Here are two more case histories that illustrate issues in the diagnosis and treatment of major depression. Alice taught me just how persistent one has to be to make the diagnosis of affective disorder and how easy it is to be thrown off by an unusual set of circumstances.

Alice was a woman in her mid-forties who was referred for admission to the university medical center where I was a first-year resident in psychiatry. She was depressed, but she had good

*L. Squires, et al., "Electroconvulsive therapy and complaints of memory dysfunction: A prospective three-year follow-up study." *British Journal of Psychiatry*, 142 (1983): 1–8.

reason to be—or so it seemed. Alice was happily married and had an eighteen-year-old daughter. Years before her depression began, her husband's elderly father had come to live in their home. He was physically ill and needed almost constant attention. He had to be helped to the bathroom, required a special diet, and could not bathe himself; in other words, Alice became a full-time nurse with one patient. What made her task much more difficult, however, was that her father-in-law was, to put it mildly, a difficult person. He was demanding to the point of being exasperating, and nothing she did seemed to please him. Food was too hot or too cold; he hated his low-salt diet and blamed Alice for being a bad cook. Nothing was right. Her husband spent long hours at his job, and though he was sympathetic, he provided little help at home either with the care of his father or with the usual housework.

Alice was from the mountains of West Virginia. She came from a simple, hardworking family and had been raised with what we might today call old-fashioned ideas. One such idea was that old folks deserved to be taken care of at home in their declining years and that it was the job of the woman of the house to provide as much care as was needed. No complaints.

The old man was chronically ill but nevertheless hung on for many years. Alice cheerfully carried out her duties for a long time. Grandpa was a tyrant whose demands ruled the household. Alice's daughter Terry grew from childhood into adolescence in a home dominated by a sick, bitter old man. Terry's one relief from the oppressive atmosphere at home was the time she spent with the next-door neighbors. Judy and Bob were a childless couple in their late thirties who had always treated Terry as an unofficial niece. They showered her with gifts at Christmas and on birthdays, took her to the movies, invited her to barbecues. Alice was glad for their interest in Terry. As Grandpa became more feeble, her time and energy were taken up more and more by his needs, and besides, Bob owned the biggest furniture store in town and so he and Judy could do things for Terry and buy her things that she otherwise might miss out on. Terry spent more and more time next door, began to stay overnight, and even went on extended vacations with Judy and Bob.

Years passed. The old man died. At last Alice could start enjoying her own family again—or so she thought.

On her eighteenth birthday, the day she was no longer a minor, Terry announced to her parents that she wanted to be legally adopted by Bob and Judy. Alice was devastated. She appealed to Bob and Judy to talk Terry out of her plan, but they said that it was Terry's decision and that they could provide for her better than Alice and her husband anyway. Alice's husband was of little help. He was so angry at Terry's announcement that he was ready to disown the girl and never speak to her again.

Alice became more and more distraught. She couldn't sleep at night; she awoke in the early morning hours and reviewed the past years again and again. "I shouldn't have let her go next door so much; I shouldn't have let her go next door so much," she repeated over and over to herself. She felt she had failed as a mother, and since her upbringing had stressed that role as the most important thing in her life, this was the most shameful failure she could know. She lost weight and looked thin and haggard. Finally she went to her family doctor to get some sleeping tablets. Her doctor noticed how depressed she looked, heard the story of Terry's leaving, and referred her to a psychiatrist. "You need to talk to somebody about all this. No wonder you feel so bad," he said. The psychiatrist saw her several times and decided that perhaps an antidepressant would help. Weeks went by; the antidepressant seemed to help a little, but Alice was still very depressed. She could think about nothing but her daughter and how she had failed as a mother. She started to be bothered by thoughts that perhaps she didn't deserve to live. The psychiatrist referred her to the university medical center for possible ECT.

Alice was admitted to my service. She looked depressed even to the untrained eye, but I had seen many patients who were much more depressed. When she told me her story I reacted as a lot of cocky trainees do, by denigrating the physician whose treatment had "failed" and who had referred her to the university. I said (to myself, thank goodness), "Don't these small-town shrinks take the time to *talk* to their patients? They see a few tears and start throwing pills at them without taking the time to see what's going on in their lives." Clearly, I thought, this was a reactive depression. The precipitant was clear, and the severity of the depression was proportional considering the facts. Certainly she had vegetative signs and anhedonia—but didn't she have good reason to? Surely a sensitive and intuitive budding psychotherapist like me was all she needed. There was nothing chemical about this depression!

I didn't see any reason to stop the antidepressant she had been taking, since she said it had helped a little. (Placebo effect, I thought!) I saw her an hour every day for therapy. After only a few days I began to doubt my hasty assessment. Alice sat hour after hour, day after day in my office, wringing her hands and repeating over and over, "I shouldn't have let her go next door; I shouldn't have let her go next door." She could talk briefly about her own past, her relationship with her husband, and other life events, but she kept returning to her own failings as a mother. Her feelings of guilt totally preoccupied her. She was stuck, almost chained, to one idea. Her mood never changed; her pained expression was as consistent from hour to hour and day to day as if she were a marble statue. Alice's unwavering distress was a clinical picture I would see again and again in patients with major depression.

Her psychiatrist had wanted her to have a course of ECT, and she was already scheduled. I had hoped to bring about a big enough change in a few days of intensive psychotherapy to persuade him to give psychotherapy another chance and perhaps avoid a long and expensive course of ECT. But I hadn't gotten any further then he, so the course of ECT was started.

As ECT began, I was astonished to see the typical signs of improvement of a major depression reponsive to ECT. Even after the first treatments, there were hours when Alice looked more relaxed and cheerful. At first this faded after the immediate posttreatment hours, as usual. But after a week there were the unmistakable signs of improvement: her handwringing became less noticeable, and smiles were more frequent. After a usual number of treatments, eight or ten, Alice was a new woman—or rather, the old Alice.

She had not completely adjusted to her daughter's moving out, of course. But she was confident that she had done the best job of raising her daughter that anyone could have done in the circumstances. She was sure that Judy and Bob would soon discover the difference between a houseguest and a daughter and grow tired of the responsibility of a full-time dependent. Terry would eventually come to realize how devoted Alice really was to her. The guilt and preoccupation were gone, and though she was certainly not happy,

Alice was freed from the total entrapment by her mood that had been so striking when she was first admitted to the hospital. She could see beyond this one event in her life and put the affair into perspective in a way she was unable to do while weighted down by her low mood and guilty feelings. She was eating normally and sleeping without sedatives. Alice was discharged from the hospital and went back to the West Virginia mountains. I received a Christmas card some months later. Alice said she was feeling her old self, and she didn't even mention her daughter.

This is a fascinating case history. I tell it often to my patients, usually to those who say they don't want to take medication because "medication won't solve my problems." Not only can the onset of an episode of affective disorder coincide with a traumatic life event, but as we have seen, a traumatic life event can precipitate an episode. I also relate it to therapists, especially nonphysicians, as an example of how we can be *too* understanding and in the psychotherapeutic search for "insight" deprive a patient of the medical intervention necessary for recovery.

In discussing the symptoms of major depression, I mentioned obsessional thoughts. Remember that an obsession is an unpleasant idea that keeps intruding into consciousness despite efforts to turn one's thoughts to something else. Alice's preoccupation with her daughter's wanting to be adopted and her self-blaming ruminations are an excellent example of this particular symptom. For many patients there is a particular theme or thought that is the earmark of their episodes of depression and does not bother them at other times. While they are depressed they can think of little else. It is amazing to see how these "mountains" shrink to their true "molehill" size as the depression lifts. When they are feeling better, patients are sometimes embarrassed to have been so troubled by a problem that seems insignificant in their normal state of mind. Often people with major depression can spot the beginning of a relapse when a particular thought or set of thoughts returns. Their change in mood is like a rainstorm coming to the desert; all kinds of dormant seeds suddenly come to life and start growing. In this case, however, the flowers are not pretty. They are usually guilty self-recriminations about unpleasant things.

Several years ago I was called to the emergency room of the hospital where I worked to see a patient who had been brought in by her family. The emergency-room physician told me the patient was a woman in her late fifties who had cancer and was very depressed.

On the way to the emergency room, walking through the musty basement halls of the hospital, I began to conjure up a picture of what she would be like. I imagined a very thin, tragically heroic woman surrounded by her grieving family, weeping softly but trying to bear up and be strong for her distraught husband and children. What I found in the examining room did not resemble my imaginings at all.

Severe depression can be a violent, wrenching condition. When Dante imagined hell, he depicted a terrifying greeting at its entrance: "All hope abandon, ye who enter here." The loss of hope is the most profound horror a person can know. This woman was suffering the torments of the damned.

Sylvia was a housewife who, a year before I saw her, had been found to have a malignant growth at the back of her throat. The growth was small, but it was invasive and inoperable. Although the oncologist had told her family she had six months to live, Sylvia had surprised everyone by continuing to do reasonably well long after her diagnosis. She had a little pain but practically no impairment in her daily functioning. This was not really surprising once you knew Sylvia. She was hardworking, ordinary, and solidly predictable, a woman of common sense and plain dealings. Cheerful, encouraging, optimistic, strong, she was the kind of person no one could imagine even getting sick, let alone dying. It was thus all the more shocking that she had become the person in the emergency room.

I saw a moaning, writhing woman on the stretcher, her husband and daughter trying ineffectively to restrain and comfort her. I learned that even though her cancer continued in remission, she had been getting increasingly depressed over the past several weeks. She had had a setback about a month earlier when it was discovered that a small tumor had spread to her lung, but she had been started on medication to stop the swelling this caused and had again been doing well. It was not in her nature to give up on

things, but her family noted a new sadness about her. She stopped
paying attention to her appearance, lost her appetite, and became
lethargic. Most worrisome, she began to expect death at any moment; she would wring her hands, sure each day would be the last.
She had nightmares about death, funerals, and graves. Then her
lethargy suddenly changed to agitation and distraction; she began
pleading, "I'm dying, take me to the hospital."

By the time I saw her in the emergency room, the depressive
process had reached its awful climax and Sylvia had crossed the
line into psychosis. "I'm dead," she moaned. "Take me to the ceme-
tary; take me to hell."

Psychiatrists use the term *delusion* to describe a persistent
false belief that is preoccupying and usually extremely distressing.
In the most severe forms of the depression of affective disorder,
delusions can occur. As in Sylvia's case, the delusions of major
depression are always—well, depressing. Severely depressed patients can become convinced they have been singled out by God
for punishment for terrible sins. (Remember guilt is a quality of
the depression of affective disorder.) Some are sure they have a fatal
disease, often a shameful one—syphilis in years gone by and more
recently AIDS. The belief that one has lost all one's money has been
called the delusion of poverty. The themes of the delusions—loss,
guilt, illness, and death—reflect the change in mood and can be
understood intuitively as arising from the abnormal mood state.
For this reason they are called mood congruent. They are in contrast
to the delusions of schizophrenia, which are more often bizarre and
do not seem to have any relation to mood. The belief that one's
phone is bugged or that neighbors are sending X rays through the
walls to harass one are examples of mood incongruent delusions;
they are upsetting, but they don't have much relation to mood.

Sylvia, naturally, was immediately admitted to the psychiatric
unit of the hospital. She was given a course of ECT and made a
dramatic recovery from her depression. She regained her cheerful,
simple "life is what you make of it" attitude and endeared herself
to other patients and staff. Before she went home Sylvia had her

husband bring a camera to the hospital and take pictures of her with all her new friends; she had heard that ECT sometimes makes you forgetful, and she wanted to remember everyone she had met and come to know. Some months later we heard that Sylvia had died at home with her family, content and cheerful to the end.

There is much we can learn from Sylvia and her psychiatric problems. Let's look at some details one by one. I left out an important point in presenting Sylvia's medical history. I didn't tell you that the medication she was given when it was discovered that her tumor had spread was prednisone. This is a preparation of a hormone produced by the human adrenal glands; when given in high doses, it can shrink certain tumors. It is one of the class of hormones and hormone derivatives called steroids. The steriods are used to treat many illnesses, for in addition to shrinking some tumor tissues, they suppress inflammation. Thus they are used in chronic inflammatory diseases such as arthritis, certain bowel diseases such as colitis, and also for lung problems such as chronic bronchitis and some cases of asthma. The steriods are powerful and effective, but they have many side effects. One is that they can cause a change in mood indistinguishable from major depression (they cause the depressive syndrome). Adding this medication to Sylvia's treatment probably is what caused her to develop psychiatric symptoms. (More on medications that can mimic mood disorders is given in chapter 6 under "Medical Causes of Mood Disorders.")

Second, and Sylvia's case makes the point even more strongly than Alice's, if the patient has the qualities of mood change and other accompanying symptoms of major depression, even if the depression seems "understandable," one should not be tricked into interpreting severe depression as merely reactive. Sylvia's family made this mistake in the early weeks of her depression; after all, she had terminal cancer and had just had a setback. Who wouldn't be depressed? If her depression had been caught earlier and properly diagnosed, it might have been treated more easily.

Third, treatment of psychiatric problems, especially affective disorder, for which such effective and safe treatments are available, should always be aggressive and persistent. It would have been rather easy to rationalize not proceeding to ECT in managing Sylvia's case. Yet when her psychiatric problem was treated, Sylvia's optimism and courage were an inspiration to all of us on the staff and certainly a comfort to her family. Her final months, of which many weeks might had been lost had medication been tried and failed, were full of life, contented, and happy.

This brings me to a discussion of the choice of medication versus ECT in treating particular patients with major depression. Let's explore the pros and cons of each: Treatment with medication is certainly simpler. Taking a couple of pills or capsules once or twice a day is quick and easy. The main problem with antidepressants is the unavoidable delay between the initiation of treatment and significant improvement in symptoms. A course of ECT more or less requires an inpatient hospital stay, with a trip to the operating room or treatment suite several times a week for two to four weeks. Most important, it requires general anesthesia for each treatment. Also, the brief periods of disorientation after the treatment can be distressing. I've already mentioned the memory problems; these are minor in the vast majority of cases but troublesome nonetheless. When trying to decide on a treatment course, I like to think of ECT as a kind of surgical procedure; it is not without risk but is clearly indicated in some cases. The decision to proceed with ECT is clear when the depression is life threatening. Patients whose nutritional status is critical need a treatment that is going to work quickly. The desperately suicidal patient is another obvious case. Patients who are distraught, sleepless, and agitated can exhaust themselves, become dehydrated, and even suffer a heart attack or stroke because of their distress. ECT can sometimes bring about significant symptom relief after one or two treatments—that is, in only a few days. When the situation is an emergency, ECT is indicated.

Although there is disagreement on the exact numbers, there is considerable evidence that antidepressant medication simply is not effective in all cases of the depression of affective disorder, and ECT is sometimes the only thing that will work. Earlier I discussed delusions—false beliefs that are very distressing but that the patient cannot be persuaded to abandon. There is some evidence that in patients who have delusional thinking as part of the symptom picture, medication alone will be ineffective and ECT will be necessary. To some extent this is an academic point; delusional patients are obviously very ill and usually need quick symptom relief, so ECT is a logical treatment choice from them anyway. Finally, ECT should of course be considered if the patient simply is not responding well to medication.

To sum up the guidelines in making this decision: Medication will work in the vast majority of patients, especially those whose symptoms are not too severe. ECT becomes the treatment of choice if an emergency exists, if adequate trials of medication have failed, and perhaps in elderly patients, for whom it seems to work especially well and quickly.

Tests for Affective Disorder

From the moment psychiatrists formulated the idea that some mood problems might have a biological basis, the search was on for a biological marker—something that could be seen or measured in the body to "make the diagnosis" of affective disorder. As we shall see in a later chapter, such a search by one psychiatrist led to one of the most valuable discoveries in the therapy of affective disorder—lithium. Was there some blood test, X ray, or brain scan that could measure the change in body chemistry in patients having an episode of affective disorder? Several tests have been developed that seemed to hold great promise. Unfortunately, none have proved valid or accurate enough to be of much practical use diagnostically.

I briefly mentioned MHPG in a previous section. MHPG stands for the dizzying chemical name of a by-product of one of the neurotransmitters, norepinephrine. (The full name for MHPG is 3-methoxy-4-hydroxyphenylglycol.) In the early seventies there was great enthusiasm for what was called the amine hypothesis of depression. Many of the neurotransmitters are classified as amines, chemical compounds that contain nitrogen. Simply put, it was thought that the depression of affective disorder might be caused by a lower than normal level of one of the amine neurotransmitters, norepinephrine. Since norepinephrine levels in the brain were thought to be correlated with levels of its by-product MHPG, and since MHPG was excreted in the urine, perhaps a diagnosis could be made by measuring MHPG levels in the urine. This line of thought became much more developed in later years; by-products of other neurotransmitters were measured in depressed and nondepressed persons, and claims were made for the diagnostic ability of several tests. For some time it was thought that perhaps MHPG tests could help pick the antidepressant that would work best for a particular patient. I've already described how frustrating this choice can be.

Unfortunately, as more and more work was done the data became more confused, not less so. Interest in MHPG has waned. Some research projects in depression still involve measuring MHPG, but everyday clinical usefulness has never materialized.*

About ten years later another laboratory evaluation emerged as a possible test for the depression of affective disorder. It was based on some observations about the way hormone levels change in people with affective disorder and is called the dexamethasone suppression test (DST). It has been known for some time that some hormones, the chemical messengers that various tissues of the body secrete to regulate the functions of other tissues, are produced with a certain rhythm and cyclicity. The most obvious example is the cycle of the "female" hormones that control menstruation. A rhythmic rise and fall of several hormones secreted by the pituitary gland at the base of the brain, as well as of the more familiar ovarian hormones estrogen and progesterone, causes the ovaries to release eggs and renews the lining of the uterus on a monthly cycle. In both men and women there is an even more striking cycle involving cortisol, a hormone secreted by the adrenal glands found above the kidney. The level of cortisol rises and falls in a daily cycle, with its lowest level measured at midnight and its peak at about 6:00 A.M.

It was discovered that in some depressed persons the normal daily rhythm of cortisol secretion did not occur. There was some of the usual rise and fall, but the adrenal glands seemed to put out an abnormally high amount of cortisol around the clock. In addition, when depressed patients were given a dose of dexamethasone, a cortisol-like drug that usually "turns off" or suppresses cortisol production temporarily in normal persons, they continued to have high levels of cortisol. The test consists of giving a dose of dexamethasone and then drawing a sample of blood when the cortisol

*Davis and Bresnahan, "Psychopharmacology in clinical psychiatry," in *American Psychiatric Association Annual Review*, 6. ed. Hales and Francis (Washington, D.C.: American Psychiatric Association Press, 1987), 160–66.

should be at its lowest point in the cycle. If the blood level was high, it was thought that one could diagnose the depression of affective disorder and that the patient should be given antidepressant medication.

The problem is that there are many cases of major depression the test does not pick up (false negative test results), and many conditions other than depression can cause a positive result (false positive test). In a healthy young person the DST will be accurate most of the time; but the risk of giving an antidepressant to a healthy young person is so low that a negative test would not preclude a trial of medication anyway. Like the MHPG tests, the DST is still useful for studying depression in various research projects, but for practical guidance in deciding whether to start a patient on antidepressants, it gives the wrong results too often to be very helpful.

Other tests are being evaluated. Many resemble the DST in that they involve hormones, since depressed patients seem to have a whole variety of alterations in hormonal functioning. Evaluations of the thyroid hormones may turn out to be useful; even growth hormone (which controls a number of functions other than growth) has been found to have abnormal levels in depression. All this work is in the early stages and is of scientific rather than practical interest at this point. So, unfortunately, there are no tests for affective disorder—at least not yet.

Unless, of course, one considers a course of ECT or a trial of medication for affective disorder to be a test. For many years psychiatrists were reluctant to just "give it a try" with medical treatment of affective disorder. To some extent this sprang from a misunderstanding of what affective disorder is. Before the discovery of today's effective medical treatments for mood disorders, almost all treatment for psychiatric disorders focused on psychotherapy, and most theories on their origin involved mechanisms and solutions that could be understood from the psychotherapeutic point of view. Vastly oversimplified, this view is that personality style, ways of coping with adversity and conflict, and the development of psychiatric symptoms are the result of life experiences, especially early childhood experiences. Psychotherapy seeks to make patients aware of how these experiences contribute to their personality and to the symptoms they are suffering and helps them to grow emotionally, develop new coping skills, and approach adversity in a more mature and effective manner.

Many believed that antidepressants, and all other psychiatric medications for that matter, simply treated symptoms without getting to the "real" cause of the problems, a cause that was essentially psychological—the result of childhood trauma, repressed unpleasant experiences, and other problems the patient would need to "work through" in psychotherapy.

This point of view is fortunately falling by the wayside. Advancements in neurochemistry indicate a biological basis for affective disorder and few believe that treatment with medication will "cover up" some deep-rooted underlying problem that will only make itself known in other ways or with other symptoms. There is really no reason not to use available treatments—especially antidepressants, which have almost no dangerous side effects—if there is any chance they may help. Such a trial is at this point the only test for affective disorder available, and it can prevent long periods of unhappiness and perhaps save a great deal of money that might be wasted on other types of treatment by nonphysicians.

This is not meant to minimize in any way the necessity of psychotherapy in treating affective disorder. On the contrary, people who are suffering from mood disorders need a tremendous amount of professional support, reassurance, and education. As they get better, most do not need weekly hour-long sessions to discuss their childhood experiences, marital relationships, and so forth, but the vast majority do need frequent visits initially to monitor their symptoms and any side effects, help them adjust to their diagnosis and treatment, and most important, to help them put all these issues into perspective and get on with their lives. Patients, especially those with mood disorders that have been untreated for a long time, may suddenly find relationships strained, develop job dissatisfaction, and even have symptoms of anxiety. Change is always painful, and even getting well is a change and can take some adjusting to. "If only I had done something about this sooner" is a comment I often hear. I'll be discussing these issues in more detail later (see "Psychotherapy" in chapter 7).

FOUR

BIPOLAR DISORDER

"Manic-Depressive Illness"

When I prescribe antidepressant medication for major depression my patients sometimes ask me, "Do I have manic-depression?" Many people have heard this term and are acquainted with the idea that "manic-depression" is a disease, a "chemical imbalance" that is treated with medication. I hope the foregoing chapters make clear that in some people depression can be the only symptom of a mood disorder and that it too is very much a disease, requiring medical treatment and responding to medication. What then is "manic-depression"?

Let me start by reviewing some of what I discussed in the first chapter, specifically the description of a good mood. I said that when people are in a good mood they are optimistic, self-assured, and confident. A good mood makes one energetic, ready for new projects and challenges, and perhaps less troubled than usual by a fear of failure. Now imagine an emotional state in which all these qualities of mood are abnormally magnified, and you will begin to understand what the manic state is like. *Manic-depression,* or more properly *manic-depressive illness*—or even more accurately *bipolar disorder,* as it is now called—is a mood disorder in which the affected person has both episodes of depression or low mood and an abnormal mood that is in some respects the opposite of depression, which is called the *manic state* or *mania*. To illustrate this disorder, I'll describe a case.

Dave is a salesman for a large insurance company; he is one of the most successful agents in his district, and the company has led him to believe that when the district manager retires in the next year or so he will be offered that position. Dave is in his early thirties, single, healthy, and fit. He lives in the same town as his parents and is close to his family. In the office Dave has a reputation as a workaholic, a high-energy person who would rather be calling on customers than going to a movie or ballgame. Nevertheless, he's well liked by his friends, customers, and co-workers.

It seemed odd, then, when John, the district manager, began to get complaints about Dave from customers. He had recently had two phone calls from policyholders complaining that Dave was "badgering" them. Dave had called them several times in the same week trying to get them to buy more insurance. One customer was furious because Dave had awakened him at 6:00 A.M. when he had said just the night before that he wasn't interested in more coverage. Dave was a good salesman, and customer relations was his specialty; he had always walked the fine line between persistence and pestering with great skill. Customer complaints about him were simply unknown.

John thought he should drop by Dave's office and pass on the complaints. Perhaps Dave had been pushing himself too hard this past month; some of the paperwork he had turned in was a little sloppy, and Dave was usually very precise in this regard. When John met with Dave he noticed the slightest change in his appearance and manner. Dave's usually meticulously organized desk was covered with papers and folders, and his shirt was wrinkled. Nevertheless, he was his energetic self, perhaps even more energetic than usual.

"You can't blame me for trying harder!" Dave replied cheerily when John mentioned the complaints. "I won't double my sales this year by giving up easily!"

"Double your sales?" John asked, "Dave, you're already the top salesman in the district. Don't burn yourself out."

"Johnny, I have a great feeling about this year. I just know I can double my sales; it's just a matter of persistence, persistence, persistence. As for the 6:00 A.M. call, well, the early bird catches the worm!"

"OK Dave, I guess I can't be too hard on you for being a good salesman. But I think you need to slow down a little. As I said, don't burn yourself out."

"Right."

John had a nagging uneasiness about their meeting, a feeling that something wasn't quite right, that there was something different about Dave. He had an intensity, a driven quality that was more than just his usual energy. And what was this "Johnny" stuff? Nobody ever called him "Johnny."

John's uneasiness was borne out the next week when he got three more customer complaints. One woman said she had felt intimidated by Dave on the phone and had agreed to buy insurance just to keep him from calling back. John went to call Dave into his office for a real meeting this time; Dave's job was in jeopardy if these complaints got to higher levels in the company. He discovered him at his desk, which was again covered with papers, files, and notebooks.

"Johnny, I'm working on something that is going to revolutionize the way this company does business. Listen to this!"

Without even waiting to hear why John had come to see him, Dave launched into a description of a scheme for selling insurance over the phone using automatic dialing machines, a scheme that was—well, crazy. It was difficult to interrupt him and get him into John's office where they could talk. John started to tell Dave to forget starting anything new and concentrate on working out his customer relations problems. Dave wanted to discuss his new marketing techniques, and their conversation started to get heated. "No wonder you're getting out of the business, Johnny; you're behind the times! You can't deal with the fact that a real innovator like me is going to take your job away from you, triple the sales of this office, and make you look like a fool. District manager is just the beginning—I'm going to run this goddamned company one day."

John had actually said very little. Dave was doing all the talking; in fact he was hoarse. Also, Dave was getting angrier by the minute and finally stormed out of the office. John tried to get him to come back, but Dave was off down the corridor like a shot, and

John let him go. He started walking back to his own office, "What's wrong?" he wondered. Was Dave drinking? Using drugs?

There was more. On the way back to his office, John picked up his mail from his secretary. There was a letter from a local bank. Dave had applied for a mortgage in the past week—a mortgage on a $500,000 home. On the application he had projected salary and commision of $1 million for the next year. Would John verify that this was possible? Dave had already put $25,000 down on the house. "God," thought John. "He must have put down all his savings and cashed in his IRA to do this."

I'll interrupt the story here, not because Dave's manic episode has reached its most severe state, but because the essential features of mania are well illustrated at this point.

As you can see, the idea that people in the manic state are simply happy while those in the depressive state are sad is not entirely accurate. As with the depression of affective disorder, the manic state of affective disorder can be defined as an abnormal change in mood, with certain accompanying peculiarities of the mood state and a change in "vegetative" functions such as sleep and energy level (see table 4). As with depression, the manic state starts in-

Table 4   Common Symptoms of the Manic State

Elevated Mood

>   Pervasive, expansive, infectious quality
>   Overconfidence, grandiosity (can become the basis for delusional thinking)
>   Sudden preoccupation with success, wealth, power, fame
>   Irritability, angry outbursts, paranoid feelings
>   Pressured socialization
>   Spending sprees, foolish investments

Vegetative Signs

>   Decreased need for sleep
>   Appetite disturbance
>   High energy, pressured speech, racing thoughts
>   Hypersexual behavior

sidiously, in many cases with a minor elevation of mood. The person becomes mildly elated, optimistic, and confident. As the clinical course goes on this "overconfidence" becomes worse, and the most striking quality of the elated mood state can be grandiosity. This can be understood as an exaggeration of the self-confidence that is usually part of a good mood. Manic people can believe they are more talented, more intelligent, more wealthy, more everything than others. This can worsen to the point where they become delusional—convinced of ideas that are impossible. In the full-blown state patients can, for example, believe they have been elected to some high political office, that they have been appointed by God for a religious mission, or even that they are God. They may become convinced that they are on the verge of great scientific discoveries, that they have developed a new economic theory that will wipe out poverty, or that they have solved the mysteries of the universe. Some become convinced that religious revelations have been made to them. Spending sprees are common, and patients sometimes borrow large sums of money or run up huge credit card bills.

The mood of the manic state has been described as expansive, and manic patients sometimes show what has been called pressured socialization—seeking out people, getting involved with new organizations (or starting new ones!), and talking to everyone in sight in a pressured, driven way. Also, their mood has been described as "infectious," meaning that just being around a manic person requires a great deal of energy and may even seem to boost one's own energy level.

Hypersexual behavior is also seen; the sex drive is abnormally heightened. Sometimes patients seek out prostitutes or otherwise lose inhibitions and engage in sexual activity that is unusual for them. One of my patients was a very quiet accountant in his forties who had never married, didn't date women, and lived at home taking care of his elderly parents. When he started to become manic he sought out homosexual encounters at local gay bars and clubs; when his mood returned to normal, he returned to his quiet but rather asexual life-style, explaining his behavior during his abnormal mood state as an aberration brought about by "mental illness." It was clear to me, however, that he had never come to terms with being sexually attracted to men and usually totally denied his sexual orientation to himself and to others. The loss of sexual inhibitions brought about by his abnormally elated mood allowed his true sexual desires to be expressed, desires he suppressed when his mood returned to normal.

In most patients the euphoria of the manic state is short-lived, and their mania soon becomes very unpleasant. Many don't get particularly euphoric at all but develop what has been called a dysphoric state. The energy level is boosted to the point where they feel pressured, driven, and in a very uncomfortable state of mind. They can be quite irritable, becoming enraged at the smallest perceived slight. Their thoughts race, their minds so speeded up that they can't talk fast enough to express them, and speech can become incoherent.

Paranoia, an unwarranted suspiciousness and the false belief that one is being persecuted, can be seen. Usually the paranoia can be understood as arising out of the grandiose mood; that is, it is mood congruent. For example, patients may believe the phone is tapped because their phone calls are so important. They may feel that others are jealous because of their special talents or great wealth or are trying to get at them because of their discoveries or religious powers.

You may think some of these symptoms don't sound so bad. More energy than usual, less need for sleep, euphoria. Couldn't everyone use a few days in this state now and then? But let's think about Dave again for a moment. He may lose his job because of his manic episode. Even if his boss is understanding, a lot of the customers he's been bothering won't be, and he's surely lost several good ones because of his harassment. He's taken all the money out of his IRA to pay for a house he can't afford. He may get his down payment back, but he probably won't recover some of the loan application costs he's already paid. And I'm not too sure the IRS would forgive his juggling with the IRA at tax time.

Sexual infidelity during such an episode may be forgiven by a spouse, but the relationship may never be quite the same. Also, with the growing prevalence of the AIDS virus, what was once considered just an indiscretion can have fatal results.

Before medications were available to end the manic state, mania had a significant mortality rate. Patients exhausted themselves and simply collapsed, dead from a heart attack, cerebral hemorrhage, or dehydration. Mania is *not* pleasant.

Another term that is sometimes applied to an abnormal mood seen in bipolar disorder is *mixed affective state*. This mood has qualities of both major depression and the manic state. Usually the irritability and driven, hyperactive energy level of mania are present, but the emotional quality is that of depression, with feelings of hopelessness and even impending doom. Separating out this mood state from mania may be artificial, since, as I state above, most of the feelings seen in the manic state are not pleasant. Mixed affective state is probably simply a severe form of mania.

The manic state of affective disorder is obviously an abnormal mental condition. It usually seems to arise out of nowhere, and the person is so changed that it is easy to conclude that something is very wrong. Mania cannot be mistaken for a normal mood state except in its earliest stages. Therefore the disease concept, that some change in brain chemistry has occurred, is easy to invoke, as John did in wondering if Dave was "on drugs." Let me emphasize here that the manic state is not just "getting carried away" or overenthusiastic about something; it is not in any way self-induced. The manic state, like the major depressive syndrome, is an expression of a change in brain chemistry. I'll discuss some ideas about what this change in chemistry may be later in this chapter.

Many patients who develop a manic state have had a prior episode of the depression of affective disorder. In some cases a single episode of bipolar disorder can have a triphasic character—that is, there are three phases to the episode. Often there is a brief period of depression that is not very severe and lasts only a few weeks or even a few days. The mood suddenly swings into a manic state that may last for several weeks, and finally depression sets in again for several weeks more. This swinging of the mood from one extreme to the other is the most striking characteristic of this form of affective disorder and led to the name given it at the turn of the century, *manic-depressive psychosis*. Today it is called *bipolar disorder*. By the way, most experts believe that affective disorder characterized by manic episodes only does not exist. Though many more people suffer from major depression than from bipolar disorder, bipolar disorder is far from rare. Most studies estimate prevalence rates at about 1 percent of the population.

So then, how do I answer my patient, about to start antidepressant medication, who asks, "Do I have manic-depressive illness?" What this question really addresses is the relation between major depression and bipolar disorder.

Another Duality

In the chapter on depression I discussed the classification of depression and introduced the terms *endogenous depression* and *reactive depression.* I now want to discuss several other terms which have been used to classify depression. At one time the terms *unipolar depression* and *bipolar depression* were used, referring respectively to mood disorders characterized by episodes of depression alone and to mood disorders characterized by both episodes of depression and episodes of the manic state in the same person. Because the term *bipolar depression* is a bit self-contradictory, it has been abandoned. The new term is simply *bipolar disorder.*

Let me pause a moment to make a very important point about the depression of affective disorder. The symptoms of depression in those with bipolar disorder are in many respects identical to the symptoms of those who have only episodes of depression, although the depressive symptoms seen in bipolar disorder tend to be more severe, and bipolar patients who become depressed often are more slowed down or "retarded" than patients with major depression. In other words, the clinical picture of depression caused by a change in brain chemistry is often virtually the same. Differentiating between major depression and bipolar disorder in depressed patients experiencing their first episode of illness is very difficult.

The latest version of the American Psychiatric Association's classification of psychiatric disorders, the *Diagnostic and Statistical Manual of Mental Disorders,* third edition, revised (the DSM-III-R) classifies the mood disorders very simply. First the manual sets out diagnostic criteria for the depression of affective disorder (an episode of which is called a major depressive episode) and the criteria for the manic state (an episode of which is a manic episode).

The DSM-III-R, then, defines the two most severe mood disorders with this simple division: major depression and bipolar disorder. At first glance it may seem somewhat arbitrary to separate out patients who have only depressions from those who have both depressive and manic episodes. However, when this separation is made and the groups are compared, there are enough differences to warrant this distinction. For example, there are subtle differences between the two groups in the age at which the first episode occurs, with bipolar disorder often beginning earlier. Major depression occurs more commonly than bipolar disorder. Major depression is much more common in women, whereas bipolar disorder is equally common in men and women. Persons with bipolar disorder often have more frequent episodes than persons with major depression. I've already mentioned the subtle differences between the symptoms of depression sometimes observed. There are also differences in the treatment of these two types of affective disorder, as we shall see later. These differences are so consistently observed that this is taken as compelling evidence that major depression and bipolar disorder are two distinct, though clearly related, mood disorders.

So what is the answer? "Do I have manic-depressive illness?" asks my patient about to start treatment for major depression. "You've got a mood disorder. You have the type of mood disorder called major depression. Manic-depressive illness, or as we call it now, bipolar disorder, is another. The relation between the two is unclear."

"Mood Swings" and Cyclothymia

In chapter 2 we saw that the depression of affective disorder can vary considerably in severity. The question naturally arises then, Can bipolar disorder also exist in more severe and less severe forms? The answer seems to be yes. Another case history will illustrate.

Tom, a thirty-year-old architect, made an appointment to see me after he had picked up a brochure on depression given out by the local community mental health center staff at a health fair in a suburban shopping mall. As he took a seat, he pulled out the little brochure and showed it to me. "This describes me perfectly!" he said, flipping through the pages. I noticed he had taken a yellow highlighter and marked the booklet as if it were a textbook. "I've known there was something wrong with me for years, but I didn't know what. Now I've discovered it! I have major depressions."

Tom was a very intense young man. He spoke quickly, concisely; listening to him reminded me of the way people read telegrams in old movies. "It started in college." Stop. "I should have seen a psychiatrist back then." Stop. "I'm sure this medication can help." Stop.

Tom clearly described episodes of the depression of affective disorder. He experienced periods of several weeks at least once or twice a year when he had such a low energy level that he stayed in bed all weekend and sometimes even took time off from work. Sometimes he seemed to lose all interest in both work and play. He would stop going to the YMCA after work, then find he had put on weight and get really down on himself, feeling fat, lazy, and good-for-nothing. He never really thought of these episodes as depression, usually shrugging them off afterward as "a virus I just couldn't shake" or "something I ate that didn't agree with me" or "cold or cloudy weather that just gets me down."

"Sometimes I get up in the morning and I know it's going to be one of those days when everybody better just steer clear of me."

"You mean you find your temper is really short some days?" I asked.

"O-o-oh yes. This is embarrassing, but I guess I need to tell you these things. One morning last week I was late getting to the bus stop, and the bus was pulling away. The driver wouldn't stop for me. I completely lost it. I was running down the street yelling and screaming. That was the worst it's ever gotten. I got this brochure just in time."

Depressed people don't go running after buses yelling at the top of their lungs. This was not simply the depression of affective disorder.

"When you have these short-tempered days, do you notice you have more energy than usual?"

"I guess you could say that. A nervous energy. I get that way too sometimes. That's when I rip through my drafting work and get a lot of routine things I've fallen behind on out of the way. I've stayed at the drafting table fifteen, twenty hours straight. It's very compulsive though; I certainly can't do anything that's at all creative."

Tom had never sought help for his mood changes; it had never even occurred to him that he might have a problem that could be helped with medication. Yet in talking to him about his past it became clear that unpredictable mood changes had been interfering with his happiness and productivity for many years. Since college he had had recurrent changes in mood and energy level lasting several days to several weeks. The changes had become severe enough in the past two years to cause him to lose time at work when he was depressed and to do embarrassing and foolish things when he was, as he called it, "nervous." He had broken up with a girlfriend because during one of his "hyper" states he had said something she felt insulted by and she wouldn't forgive him. Yet the mood swings had never become terribly severe. Because they were not extreme and because they always went away in a few days or weeks at the most, he could rationalize the symptoms as being caused by some outside agent or event—a cold virus, a tight deadline at work, losing the car keys, or even the old cliché about getting up on the wrong side of the bed.

Tom was suffering from cyclothymia. *Thymos* is a Greek word meaning mind, but it has come to be used as a root in psychiatry refering to mood. (Remember, dysthymia refers to depressed mood, *dys-* meaning bad.) The prefix *cyclo-* means just what you'd think: cycling.

Cyclothymia is essentially defined as a less severe form of bipolar disorder. The depressive periods are not serious enough to be called major depressive episodes, and the manic like states are not extreme enough to be called mania. There is even a term for this not-quite-manic state: *hypomania (hypo-* meaning below or less). It may appear arbitrary to consider cyclothymia a separate disorder from bipolar disorder. I agree, and so do many other experts in the field of affective disorder. It is clear that many people who are said to have cyclothymia will go on to develop a full-blown major depressive or manic episode and then will meet the DSM-III-R criteria for bipolar disorder. Another compelling bit of evidence linking cyclothymia and bipolar disorder is that the same treatment, the medication lithium, is effective for both.

Another aside about the classification of bipolar disorders: in some research publications you may read about "bipolar I" and bipolar II." Simply put, bipolar I patients have a clear history of both major depressive episodes and manic episodes, whereas bipolar II patients have major depressive episodes and very mild manic or hypomanic symptoms. Not everyone agrees that this distinction is clinically useful; it doesn't change the way these patients are treated for their disorder. At this point the distinction is used mainly by researchers studying the genetics—that is, the inheritance patterns—of affective disorder. But as more treatment options become available and as these distinctions are better understood, bipolar I and bipolar II may become more important concepts.

The Chemistry of Bipolar Disorder

What can neurochemistry tell us about bipolar disorder? Are there any findings that will help us understand the relation between bipolar disorder and major depression? Unfortunately, the neurochemistry of bipolar disorder is even more obscure than that of major depression. In the depression of affective disorder, the almost accidental discovery of an effective treatment led to some theories about the neurochemical basis of the disease because the treatment's effect on the brain chemistry could be measured.

The discovery of a treatment for bipolar disorder was also completely accidental, but as with many other mysterious but effective treatments in medicine (such as that other treatment of affective disorder, electroconvulsive therapy), we've discovered over the years by trial and error how to use the drug to treat the disorder. We know what dosage is needed and what the side effects are. Nevertheless, the effect lithium has on the brain is almost completely unknown.

Given that the symptoms of major depression seem to occur when there is a relative deficiency of amines such as norepinephrine, doesn't it make sense that the manic state might be caused by an excess of these substances in the brain? Again, investigating neurotransmitter levels is extremely difficult, but some theories have emerged to explain the clinical facts. One of the neurotransmitters implicated recently in mood disorders is acetylcholine. (Remember the anticholinergic side effects of antidepressants? See "Antidepressants" in chapter 3.) The thinking is that a high acetylcholine level or activity is associated with symptoms of depression and a low level with the manic state. This might explain why many an-

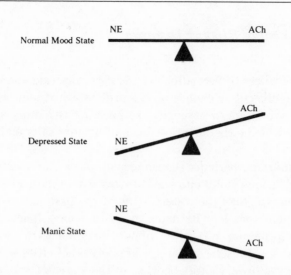

Figure 3   Neurotransmitter activity in mood states of bipolar disorder.
NE = Norepinephrine   ACh = Acetylcholine

tidepressant medications have anticholinergic effects. There may even be a link to the amine neurotransmitters like norepinephrine in that a kind of balance of the two systems is necessary for normal mood and changes in this balance can produce both of the mood syndromes of bipolar disorder (see fig. 3).

As we will see in the next section, one medication, lithium, is used to treat both the depressed and the manic phases of bipolar disorder. How can this be? How can one medication treat such different clinical states? Even more basic a question is, How can one illness have two completely opposite sets of symptoms? The answer may be that the basic defect in bipolar disorder is not in the absolute level of the neurotransmitters we have been talking about but rather in the mechanism that determines their balance (the little triangle in fig. 3), and that lithium works at this point rather than directly on the levels of the neurotransmitters. (If this seems confusing, don't worry. In the last section, after I've said a lot more about mood disorders and their treatment, I'll come back to this concept, which may be a little obscure at this point.)

The Treatment of Bipolar Disorder

Lithium

"The Three Princes of Serendip" is a Persian fairy tale about finding valuable objects by chance on a journey toward another goal.
No discovery in modern psychiatry so parallels this story as does
the discovery of the therapeutic effects of lithium salts on bipolar
disorder.

For hundreds, perhaps thousands, of years Europeans have
traveled to various small cities and towns where natural mineral
springs occur to "take the waters." One of the first such towns to
become popular has lent its name to all that have followed. Spa
is a mountain hamlet in Belgium, about thirty miles from the German border. Spa, Bath in England, and many other cities with such
natural springs drew visitors because of the water's reputed healing properties and developed into resorts. All kinds of therapeutic
effects were ascribed to various spring waters, which were bathed
in, drunk, used in massages, and formulated into elixers, teas, oint-
ments, and muds. As medical science grew more sophisticated in
the nineteenth century, it was slowly realized that many of the
illnesses the therapeutic waters were said to ameliorate were those
that were chronic but somewhat variable in their course. Illnesses
like arthritis and emphysema, for example, tend to cause symptoms
for many years but show spontaneous periods of remission, usually
followed by relapse. The "therapeutic" effect of spa waters began
to look more and more like the result of rest, good food, lots of
attention, the placebo effect, and a bit of good timing. Nevertheless,
chemists began sampling the spring waters to see what was in them.

One of the chemicals they found was lithium. Lithium is an
element, a single kind of atom, and is chemically grouped with sodium and potassium, with which it shares many characteristics. In
valiant attempts to duplicate and possibly enhance the effects of
spa waters, lithium was administered to patients with epilepsy,
diabetes, and gout. Though results were uniformly disappointing,
lithium was formulated into compounds suitable for medical use.
But like imipramine years later, these lithium compounds were put
on the shelf and forgotten.

In the 1940s the biology of salt and water balance in the body
was being investigated. Researchers discovered that restricting salt

intake was beneficial in certain medical problems where the body was impaired in its ability to excrete excess salt and water—conditions such as congestive heart failure, where water can build up in the lungs with fatal results. (Table salt consists of a sodium ion and a chlorine ion chemically bound together to form the compound sodium chloride; it is the sodium ion that is crucial to water balance in the body.) But low-sodium diets are extremely unpalatable, and it was (and still is) difficult to get patients to stick to them. The search was on for a salt substitute to flavor low-sodium foods.

Lithium, which is closely related to sodium, was pulled off the shelf, and various lithium compounds were tried as salt substitutes. The result were disastrous; lithium was found to be toxic in surprisingly small concentrations. Even worse, patients with impaired sodium excretion also were impaired in their lithium excretion and were thus setup for lithium toxicity. Several deaths were reported. Lithium was put back up on the shelf—way back in the corner of the top shelf!

In 1949 John Cade, an Australian psychiatrist, was investigating the manic state. Specifically, he was looking for a biological marker—some abnormal chemical level or measurable change in functioning that one could use to test for the disorder. Cade analyzed the urine of manic patients hoping to find some "toxin" that might signal this abnormality of mood and possibly lead to a test or even a treatment. He became convinced that the "toxin" would be a compound similar to uric acid, a by-product of protein breakdown that is a normal chemical in urine. Cade needed a form of uric acid that dissolved easily in water, and he picked lithium urate. This almost completely arbitrary choice was the first gift from the Persian princes of Serendip.

In the course of his investigations Cade injected lithium urate into laboratory guinea pigs, and he noticed that the animals became lethargic. Further experiments revealed that it was the lithium, not the urate, that induced the lethargy. I've always thought the poor little guinea pigs probably slowed down because of lithium toxicity, but Cade at first thought he had discovered a new sedative. This erroneous conclusion was the second serendipitous event. Cade tried out his new sedative in some manic patients. The results were astonishing. Although early studies were flawed in their methods, an 80 percent favorable response rate was reported.

Now, reporting a therapeutic use for lithium was a little like reporting a beneficial effect for Agent Orange would be today. Lithium had such a bad reputation that it was years before the results were noticed. It was due largely to the perseverance of a Danish psychiatrist, Morgans Schou, that any work at all was done. Schou was convinced of lithium's efficacy in treating bipolar disorder and continued to experiment with it. In 1954 he published a landmark study, "The Treatment of Manic Psychoses by the Administration of Lithium Salts," which clearly indicated that giving lithium would make the racing thoughts, agitation, and hyperactivity of the manic state gradually disappear. When the lithium was stopped, however, the symptoms returned "unless the manic phase had spontaneously subsided in the meantime."

In 1967 another paper indicated an even more valuable use for this new medication. The paper was called "Lithium as a Prophylactic Agent," and Dr. Schou was a coauthor. "Prophylactic" can be defined as preventive, and this paper showed that continuing lithium even after the resolution of the manic symptoms could prevent repeat episodes of either the manic state *or* depression. Lithium was found to have a specific action against bipolar disorder; it treated the acute symptoms and in many cases prevented symptoms from coming back for as long as the patient took it.

The prophylactic effect of lithium was at first strongly resisted. An article titled "Prophylactic Lithium, Another Therapeutic Myth?" appeared in a leading British medical journal as recently as 1968. As further studies were done, however, this effect was verified again and again. Yet it was not until 1970 that lithium became widely used in the United States. Thus American psychiatry has had less than twenty years' experience with this medication.

Unlike the antidepressants, which can be effective at a relatively wide range of doses and blood levels, lithium is effective in almost all bipolar patients only when a particular level is reached in the body. Because lithium can be toxic at levels not much higher than the level at which it is therapeutic, regular blood tests are required to make sure the patient is getting enough to be effective but not so much as to risk toxicity. It usually takes several weeks to find the dose necessary to attain a blood level in the therapeutic range. Sometimes, when the patient is having severe symptoms and the psychiatrist wants to get to the therapeutic level of lithium as soon as possible, the tests may be repeated several times a week. the correct dose is ascertained, regular blood tests are still necessary because changes in body weight, addition of medicines for other problems, and other factors can affect the lithium level.

The therapeutic range for lithium has been determined through clinical trials in which blood tests were always done twelve hours after the last dose of the medication. For this reason it is important that when a blood test is necessary patients try to be in the laboratory twelve hours after their own latest dose of medication. Since most people take a bedtime dose at about 11:00 P.M., it's usually relatively easy to put one's "A.M." dose in pocket or purse instead of taking it and to drop by the clinic or laboratory in late morning for the blood test, taking the "skipped" morning dose on the way out. This timing is very important; a blood test taken too long or short a time after the last dose will give inaccurate information, and erroneous changes in dosage may be made.

Lithium does have a number of side effects that are more uncomfortable than dangerous (see table 5). Because lithium is so closely related to sodium, the body handles it much the same way—that is, excretes it through the kidneys. Starting on lithium is simi-

Table 5   Lithium Side Effects

Short Term (Temporary)

    Increased thirst and urination
    Water retention (especially in women)

Ongoing Side Effects

    Gastrointestinal tract irritation (nausea, diarrhea; often
       treatable)
    Birth defect potential
    Tremor (dose related and also treatable)
    Concentration and memory problems (dose related)

Long Term

    Kidney problems (urine concentration problems causing exces-
       sive thirst and urination)
    Thyroid problems

lar to raising salt intake; many patients notice an increase in thirst and urination. Some people, especially women, experience water retention causing puffy fingers or ankles. The body seems to adjust quickly to the new salt/water balance, though, and this problem often subsides. It is very important not to start on a diuretic medication while taking lithium. (Diuretics, also commonly known as "water pills," increase urine production and are used to treat high blood pressure and other medical problems.) Diuretics change the way the kidneys excrete sodium (and therefore lithium), and some can cause lithium toxicity. Patients on lithium can take diuretics, but the dose may require adjustment; this should reinforce the need to tell *all* doctors about *all* the medication one is taking.

Lithium is somewhat irritating to the stomach and digestive tract, and some patients have nausea or diarrhea when they start taking it. The nausea can usually be avoided by taking the medication immediately before or after meals so that there is food in the stomach. Also, there are slow-release forms of lithium that may help with the gastrointestinal side effects.

Another common side effect is a slight tremor or shaking, especially of the hands. This tremor can get worse with anxiety or nervousness; in fact, many people notice it only at such times. If this side effect is a problem, there are medications (the beta-blockers) that can lessen it. In my experience they are usually not necessary.

Some patients report that when they are taking lithium their concentration and memory are not as efficient as usual. There have been reports of people who feel they are less creative, and there is some evidence that initiative and speed of performance on some psychological tests are dulled. Like the memory effects of ECT, these subtle changes are difficult to measure. Nevertheless, there probably are real changes in cognitive ("thinking") efficiency in some people. However, these effects seem dose related; that is, they subside if the lithium dose is lowered.

✳Lithium, unlike antidepressants, can cause long-term problems in patients who take it for extended periods. Taking lithium for a long time, usually many years, can affect the urine concentrating function of the kidneys and also can suppress thyroid gland functioning. Because of these potential side effects, blood tests are done every year or so to be sure these problems are not occurring.

The tests are only a precaution, and most people can take lithium for years at a time with no problems at all. Lithium has caused very serious cardiac birth defects, so women in the childbearing years must practice birth control while taking lithium.

Because toxic levels are so close to therapeutic levels, patients taking lithium must be familiar with the symptoms of lithium poisoning (see table 6). The most common and earliest signs are the symptoms experienced by Cade's guinea pigs—lethargy and fatigue. Dizziness, muscle weakness, slurred speech, and unsteady walk are signs of advancing toxicity and warrant a trip to the emergency room. Those taking lithium should be careful not to get dehydrated in hot weather, since this concentrates the lithium in their bodies. Patients sometimes ask if they should drink extra water or take salt tablets. This is really unnecessary because the body has a natural mechanism to make sure it has enough water: the thirst reflex. I tell my patients to drink when they are thirsty and maybe drink a bit extra for good measure, especially in hot weather. More than this is not necessary.

Another point: like the antidepressants, lithium usually takes several weeks at therapeutic levels to have its effect on abnormal mood states.

All these blood tests, toxicity, birth defects—it may seem that lithium is a lot of trouble. The patients who benefit from it will tell you differently. For those with bipolar disorder, the benefit is obvious. These patients' changes of mood and behavior can be so serious that they must be hospitalized. Sometimes the episodes can recur every few years or even more often. A medication that can

Table 6 Symptoms of Lithium Toxicity

Fatigue and lethargy
Clouded thinking and impaired concentration
Severe nausea and vomiting
Dizziness
Muscle weakness
Slurred speech
Unsteady walk

treat and thus shorten an episode of bipolar disorder and prevent future episodes thus makes the difference between a normal life and spending years in a hospital, as happened to many patients with bipolar disorder before there were effective medications.

Patients with less severe mood swings also benefit tremendously from lithium therapy. "My life is predictable for the first time in years," one of my patients with cyclothymia told me. "Before I started taking lithium, I never knew how I would feel when I got up in the morning. It was impossible to plan anything. Vacations had to be canceled because I'd wake up so depressed on the day we were to leave." Another said to me several months after starting lithium, "I feel like I always thought I was supposed to but never could. My husband told me that if I were any more normal he wouldn't know how to act around me anymore." It's often only after lithium therapy begins that patients and their families realize that for years the rhythm of their lives had danced to the syncopated beat of unpredictable mood swings.

Antidepressants and Bipolar Disorder

In Roland Kuhn's original paper on the use of imipramine in depression he noted that "in individuals who are predisposed, it may give rise to a somewhat manic-like or even manic state." He did not comment on, and probably did not realize, what this predisposition was but only reassured readers that imipramine was not a "euphoriant" and did not lead to addiction. The "predisposed" individuals Kuhn noted had bipolar disorder.

It is very clear now that antidepressants can precipitate a manic episode in persons with bipolar disorder. That they do not do so in everyone with affective disorder seems to indicate another fundamental difference between major depression and bipolar disorder. Not everyone seems to have the "chemistry" necessary to become manic, but in those who do a manic state can be induced by antidepressants.

For many years this fact was noted but did not much affect how antidepressants were used. People with symptoms of major depression were treated with antidepressants, and if they later turned out to have bipolar disorder, they could just be switched to lithium and everything would be set right. To sort out whether people with symptoms of the depression of affective disorder as their first episodes of illness had major depression or were in the depressed phase of bipolar disorder was thought to be a more or less academic exercise. There is some evidence now, however, that patients with bipolar disorder who take antidepressants can develop manic states that are more difficult to treat, and it has even been suggested that in some people antidepressants precipitate a switch to a more severe "rapid-cycling" bipolar illness and they may have more frequent episodes of illness. This last point is somewhat controversial, but a number of studies have shown that antidepressants can destabilize the mood for many weeks.

Clearly, then, it seems prudent to avoid starting antidepressants in depressed patients who may have bipolar disorder. How is this possible if the patient has never had a manic episode? One clue is a family history of bipolar disorder; we'll see later that bipolar disorder has a rather strong hereditary component, and this form of affective disorder seems to run true from one generation to the next and between closely related persons. Also, most persons with bipolar disorder have had symptoms of unstable mood states for years before they have an episode severe enough to bring them to a psychiatrist. Often a history of hypomania precedes the first severe episode of bipolar disorder, even if that episode is a depressed one. I alluded to this pattern in discussing cyclothymia. It may be that people who meet the diagnostic criteria for cyclothymia simply have sought treatment earlier in the course of their illness than those who are diagnosed as having bipolar disorder at the time of their first episode.

Other Treatments of Bipolar Disorder

TRANQUILIZING MEDICATIONS

Severe mania is a dangerous condition; as I stated above, it used to have a significant mortality rate. Some manic patients can be highly aggressive and even violent. Like suicidal depression, this is truly a psychiatric emergency.

Because lithium takes days or even weeks to work, most patients with mania need a medication to slow them down and decrease their agitation and hyperactivity until lithium achieves its therapeutic effect. Antipsychotic medication, the type originally found useful in schizophrenia, works very well for this purpose.

Some studies have even suggested that antipsychotic medication has a specific "antimanic" effect. Others seem to indicate that antipsychotics treat only some of the hyperactivity of mania and that lithium is necessary to treat the entire complex of symptoms. Many patients are put on both lithium and an antipsychotic medication when they are very sick, and as the lithium begins to work the antipsychotic is gradually tapered off in dosage and eventually discontinued. Thus antipsychotics are used in mania in much the same way as they are in severe depression: as *symptomatic* treatment. (For a discussion of the use of antipsychotic medications in severe depression see "Tranquilizing Medications" in chapter 3.)

ANTICONVULSANT MEDICATIONS

Another class of medications that is being found helpful in mania includes a number of drugs that have been used for years to treat epileptic disorders. The first was carbamazepine (Tegretol), which has been used to treat petit mal seizures. Other antiepileptic drugs being used in treating mania are valproic acid and more recently clonazepam, a drug related to diazepam (Valium). These drugs were first tried after a theory developed that mania is due to an uncontrolled discharge of the electrical activity of the theoretical "mood system" in the brain. Various advantages have been claimed for the anticonvulsants over the more widely used drugs. Carbamazepine is said to work better in patients who have "rapid-cycling" bipolar disorder, that is, who have very frequent episodes and whose symptoms sometimes are resistant to lithium therapy. Other drugs have the advantage of being less toxic than lithium or having fewer side effects. Our experience in using these drugs in mania is growing, and though none seems as consistently effective as lithium, it may be that we don't yet know which patients they work best for. Also, none have been proved to have a prophylactic effect— but it took a number of years for this added advantage to be proved for lithium. What is important is that a whole new class of drugs has been found useful in bipolar disorder, and this will undoubtedly lead to the development of new and even better medications.

ELECTROCONVULSIVE THERAPY

Before antipsychotics and lithium were known, ECT was used to treat mania. It is still used for this purpose in some patients and

it may work even faster than antipsychotic medication while producing the same specific effect as lithium on all manic symptoms—
the best of both worlds. Some experts in the field of affective disorder
now feel that ECT is underutilized as a treatment for acute mania,
and it may become more widely used for this prupose in the future.
I find it fascinating that both ECT, a treatment that causes seizures
and anticonvulsants used to prevent seizures, can be effective treatments for the manic state. No one knows why this should be. It
only serves to remind us how mysterious and complicated an illness affective disorder is.

Length of Treatment in Bipolar Disorders

The issue of how long to take medication is much more difficult
to address for bipolar disorder than for major depression. In major
depression, since the periods of remission can be much longer than
the periods of relapse, it generally has made sense to recommend
that patients take their antidepressant for the usual length of time
of a major depressive episode, six to eighteen months. (See chapter
3 for a more complete discussion of this issue.)

In bipolar disorder, however, episodes of illness generally occur
much more often—every several years, yearly, or even several times
a year. In addition, there is some evidence that episodes are more
frequent as one gets older. At one time it was recommended that
in treating the first episode of the manic state lithium be prescribed
only for several months and then discontinued. Not many clinicians
follow this plan anymore, however, because as we gain more and
more experience in diagnosing and treating bipolar disorder (remember that lithium has been widely used in this country for less
than twenty years), it has become clear that the benefits of treatment
far outweigh the risks for most patients. Some clinicians are re-
commending that once a clear diagnosis of bipolar disorder has been
made, medication be continued more or less indefinitely. Which
group is right?

Clearly, a patient who is having relapses several times a year
will want to take medication continuously. But how about the person who has had only two episodes, say five years apart? Should
someone take medication continuously for a problem that may not
come back for five more years? The key word in that sentence is

"may." Although some patients have a course of illness with regular cycles, many do not. Remember also that the episodes seem to become more frequent as time goes on.

Some work is being done to treat bipolar patients with doses of lithium that are changed over time according to patients' mood symptoms. Some sophisticated treatment methods attempt to measure mood regularly and raise and lower the dose of lithium accordingly. Some patients do well on an almost subtherapeutic lithium dose most of the time, and the dose can be raised at times when they are vulnerable to developing symptoms.

I suppose that in the final analysis how long to take medication is something only the affected person can answer, and it basically boils down to an even more difficult question: How important is it to me not to have another episode of illness? It is very clear that the most effective action one can take to prevent an episode of bipolar disorder is to take medication. Whether preventing an episode is worth taking the medication, having the necessary blood tests, using birth control during the childbearing years, and so forth, is a very personal decision. What is important is that it be an informed decision, made after careful consideration of the available facts.

Some of the most severely impaired and psychiatrically handicapped persons I have ever come in contact with were a few patients I saw while doing my training in psychiatry who did not take their diagnosis of bipolar disorder seriously. They would stop taking their medication almost as soon as they recovered from an episode of illness. I would be called to see them in the emergency room again and again over a period of years and could tell from their medical records that many psychiatric staff members before me had also seen them again and again. It seemed that these patients would stop taking medication almost willfully, when they got angry at their spouses or during some crisis at home. They appeared to use their manic state as a "drug" with which to escape some unpleasant reality. I would read through their charts and find that as episode after episode of mania occurred their employers, their friends, and sometimes even their families had lost patience and just dropped out of their lives. I saw women whose adult children would not even visit them in the hospital. In the worst cases even the hospital staff retreated into a sort of cynicism, treating the patients almost as naughty children when they got ill again, the whole effort to treat their illness degenerating into a silly, pathetic farce. Fortunately such cases are rare.

I relate this story not to frighten anyone—certainly not to intimidate anyone into meekly following doctor's orders and not asking questions—but rather to make the point that every episode of bipolar disorder has consequences and that sometimes the consequences are impossible to predict. When treatment begins soon after an episode the symptoms may resolve quickly. One problem with this, however, is that the first mood symptom may be a slight euphoria, and it is difficult to convince someone who is feeling *better* than usual of the need to take medication. Another problem is that the symptoms in bipolar disorder sometimes advance very quickly, and it may be difficult to avoid hospitalizing patients who get sick rapidly. Mania (or severe depression) can be a real emergency, and emergency decisions by family members and even psychiatrists may lack the needed careful consideration.

Instead of, Why should I continue taking medication indefinitely? perhaps those with bipolar disorder should ask themselves, Why *shouldn't* I continue taking medication indefinitely? (More on this issue is discussed under "Relapse" in chapter 7.)

PART TWO

Variations, Causes, and Connections

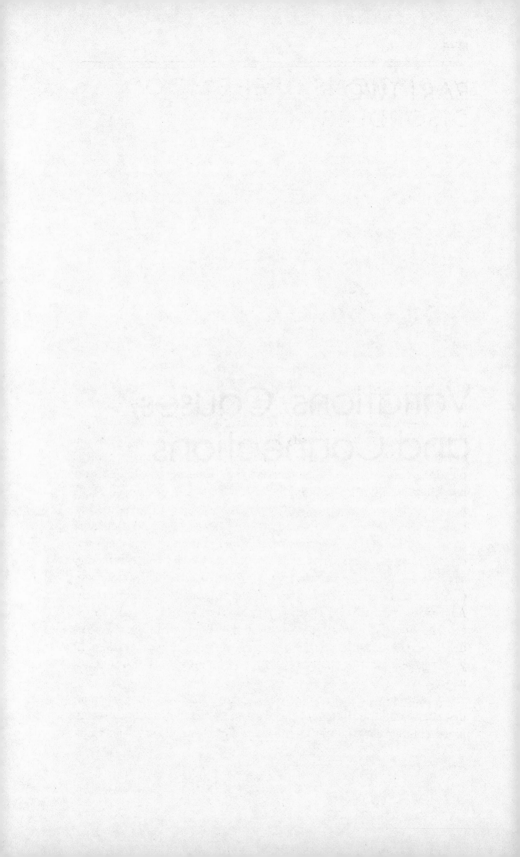

FIVE

VARIATIONS OF THE MOOD DISORDERS

The mood disorders, especially major depression, have many symptoms besides a change in mood. I've discussed many of these in the chapters on depression and bipolar disorder. Changes in appetite and sleep, energy, activity levels, and concentration are some of the symptoms, and in some people they may dominate the clinical picture or at least be so prominent that other types of illnesses, usually more familiar or more "medical" ones, are diagnosed. Also, mood disorders are very commonly seen in relation to certain other biological events and may seem causally related. The relationships of mood disorders to the menstrual cycle and to a common brain disorder, cerebrovascular accident or stroke, have been extensively studied by neuropsychiatrists, and this study has added much to our knowledge about the possible biological basis of mood disorders. Also, since more women than men suffer symptoms of mood disorders and because stroke affects so many people each year, I shall describe these relationships in some detail. Mood disorders in young people and in the elderly have some special characteristics as well.

I want to discuss the newly recognized relation between mood disorders and the change of the seasons, as well as the long-recognized connection between depression and chronic pain. The study of these variations has added tremendously to our knowledge about the biological basis of mood, and I shall present some new theories about mood disorders. Finally, I'll discuss the relation between mood disorders and panic attacks (or panic disorder), which also sheds light on the basis of all the mood disorders.

This chapter will deal with some "subtypes" of affective disorder that are especially likely to be called something else, "explained away," or missed altogether by the affected person, family members, and even doctors.

Major Depression in the Elderly

"Your mother has Alzheimer's disease. It's an incurable, deteriorating disease that causes progressive loss of thinking capacity. I suggest you start looking for a nursing home." Can a more terrible pronouncement be imagined? To see a loved one withering away, mind and body gradually failing until death is a welcome release? Becoming a pathetic shell of a person who does not recognize anyone and is bedridden, incontinent, and incoherent? And yet there is another illness that can mimic all the symptoms of Alzheimer's disease. It is major depression—and as you know by now, major depression is easily treatable.

Pearl is sixty-eight years old, a retired executive secretary who worked for a large retailer. She had been referred to me by her internist, who told me she was showing memory loss and other signs of intellectual deterioration. "She's really taken this hard. So has the family. I'm going to send them all over to your office for some counseling."

Pearl and her two daughters came into my office and sat down. "We need your advice, Doctor. We want to know what we can do for Mother—how best to help her."

Pearl sat in the middle of my small sofa between her two daughters. Both daughters sat on the edge of the cushion, their knees pointing toward the center and almost touching their mothers'. One woman held her mother's hand and looked over at her while the other watched me as she spoke. They reminded me of a triptych by some Renaissance painter, only instead of a Madonna

or crucified Christ as the center panel, this altarpiece was dominated by the figure of Despair.

Pearl was a handsome, almost stately, woman. One would be
tempted to call her robust, but her posture and expression radiat-
ed anything but health. Her skin was pale, almost sallow, her
hands were crossed in her lap like useless, heavy things, and her
shoulders drooped. Her eyes were downcast, her brow furrowed,
her mouth fixed in a deep frown. She sat motionless.

"How did your mother's difficulties begin?" I asked.

"Mother always hosts a big family dinner the first night of
Passover, and since Daddy passed away I've helped her with some
of the cooking. I went over a few weeks ahead to start planning
and found her like this." She looked forlornly at her mother.

"Can you tell me what was different?"

She turned back to me with a look of surprise, as if to say,
"What's the matter with you? Can't you see how terrible she looks?"
I tried to respond to this unstated question. "I want to know exactly what changes have occurred so I can know how best to help
your mother and you."

"Well, she was sitting in her apartment with the lights out and
the television on, but she wasn't even aware of what she was
watching. She looked like she was in a daze, just staring. Just like
this." She looked at Pearl again and then said, "I asked her,
'Mother, weren't you expecting me? Don't you remember that I was
coming over to start getting ready for Passover?' 'I can't remember
anything anymore,' she said. 'I've forgotten all the recipes anyway.'
Doctor," her voice lowered almost to a whisper, "sometimes she
doesn't even know what day it is."

"Mrs. Feldman, tell me about your memory problems."

"My memory is completely gone, Doctor," said Pearl, not even
looking up from the floor. "I don't see how you can help me; I'll
never be the same again."

"Mother, Dr. Leeds is your medical doctor. He is going to
help with your memory. This doctor will help you with your
depression."

I began asking Pearl some questions to test her memory and
thinking. "I'm going to say the names of three ordinary objects for
you, Mrs. Feldman. I want you to remember them for a few moments, and later I'll ask you to repeat them."

"I'll try."

I named the objects and then asked, "Can you subtract seven from one hundred for me? Then subtract seven from that number, and keep subtracting sevens until I tell you to stop."

"I can't; I just can't think clearly. My mind's a blank."

"I want you to try."

She sighed deeply. "Ninety-three." She was silent. The quiet daughters looked away, pained. "That's all. That's all I can do."

"OK. That's tricky, isn't it? Don't be discouraged. Can you remember those three objects?"

Pearl's brow became even more furrowed; her glance wandered about the room as if searching for the answers printed on the diplomas on the wall or the spines of the books on the shelves. Then she looked down at the floor again. "I can't remember. I told you my memory was gone."

"How has your mood been, Mrs. Feldman?"

"Terrible. How would you feel if you couldn't think, couldn't remember?"

"How has your sleeping been?"

"I toss and turn all night; I can't rest. I'm losing my mind, aren't I, Doctor? That's why Dr. Leeds sent me over here, isn't it? I should be put away, just put away in an institution."

"No, no, Mrs. Feldman; you don't need to worry about that," I replied. I leaned over and took her hand, "I'm confident that we're going to get you better."

I asked Pearl to step into the waiting room so I could talk to her daughters alone for a moment. "I want to put your mother into the hospital so we can be more aggressive in treating her depression."

"Well, if you think it's a good idea, Doctor. Can't you do some counseling or prescribe medication for her as an outpatient, though? Mother is frightened of hospitals. She could stay with one of us until she's feeling better."

"I may want to give her electroconvulsive treatments, and she would need to be in the hospital for that."

"Shock treatments! Doctor, my mother's not crazy!"

I saw I had a lot of educating to do, but I knew they would thank me in the end.

The collection of symptoms and findings typical of Alzheimer's disease is actually seen in many different conditions. Memory loss, loss of the ability to concentrate, disorientation—for example, not knowing what day it is—these are all symptoms of the psychiatric syndrome known as dementia. The demented patient is perfectly alert but experiences a decline in all intellectual functions. Dementia is usually progressive and often irreversible. But not always.

Dementia can be seen in a number of brain diseases such as Parkinson's disease or repeated strokes; even brain injury from an automobile accident can cause the syndrome. One of the commonest causes of dementia in the elderly is Alzheimer's disease, now thought to be secondary to the degeneration of a single brain center.

As the field of geriatric medicine has developed, it has become clear that many conditions often dismissed as "normal" concomitants of aging are not normal at all but are due to disease processes. It has also become clear that many of these diseases are treatable, thus making it all the more important that the physician look for them in evaluating the elderly patient. "Senility" is not normal in the elderly, and society's tendency to regard it as such is a subtle form of prejudice that has been called ageism. An even more subtle form of ageism is the tendency to make a diagnosis of "Alzheimer's disease" in every elderly person with symptoms of dementia and to write off the dementia syndrome as incurable.

As the field of geriatric psychiatry developed, the term *pseudodementia of depression* came into being to describe a condition often seen in elderly persons suffering from major depression. It was noted that the elderly depressed often have a decline in intellectual functioning that looks exactly like dementia. In fact some experts believe that the changes in brain chemistry that occur in major depression slow down the brain's functioning exactly like other dementing illnesses. Therefore in more and more articles in the professional journals the "pseudo" is being dropped and the memory problems, confusion, and concentration problems are being called simply the dementia syndrome of depression.

Often the decline in memory has qualities that specifically indicate the dementia syndrome of depression rather than dementia from another cause. Patients with this syndrome are usually extremely distressed by their deficits in intellectual functioning. This is in contrast to the picture usually seen in patients with Alzheimer's disease, who are sometimes unaware of their memory problems in the early stages and often attempt to make light of them or cover them up. Depressed patients, on the other hand, seem to dwell on their memory problems and, like Pearl, see every missed answer as confirmation of their "hopeless" condition.

ECT seems to be particularly effective in this syndrome. It works quickly and effectively, and it also has a diagnostic use. If an elderly person is showing symptoms of dementia and also of major depression, a single ECT treatment can sometimes sort out the diagnosis. Remember I said earlier that persons with brain injury were especially prone to prolonged confusion following ECT treatments. If someone has Alzheimer's disease, ECT will make the confusion much worse (temporarily); in those with the dementia syndrome of depression, ECT will make it a bit better.

The need to make this differentiation is, I hope, obvious. If the diagnosis of major depression is missed, there is the risk that the elderly patient will be written off as suffering from an incurable disease and simply sent to a nursing home.

Major depression seems to present a slightly different symptom picture in the elderly in other ways as well. The dementia syndrome of depression is one such variation. Another prominent feature in older individuals is hypochondriasis, a preoccupation with physical symptoms that sometimes grows into the conviction that one is suffering from some terrible illness. More often, the patient just seems to have one minor physical complaint after another for which no serious underlying cause can be found. Patients report physical symptoms such as vague pains, nausea, tiredness, or simply feeling "sick." It is important, of course, that anyone who has physical symptoms be evaluated for physical causes. But an older person who complains of many vague physical symptoms for which little or no basis can be found and who seems chronically upset and unhappy should be evaluated for major depression.

I have had patients referred to me by doctors who say they have given them "the million-dollar workup" for such problems. Having done every conceivable diagnostic procedure—some very expensive and even dangerous—they make a referral to a psychiatrist as a "last resort." How much time, money, and suffering might be saved by considering the diagnosis of major depression earlier on!

Another issue in evaluating depression in the elderly is the tendency to assume that depression is an expected concomitant of growing old. Persons over sixty or so are often beset by losses. Spouse, siblings, and friends may die, sometimes one after another in a short period. There is often loss associated with illness and physical incapacitation. These losses inevitably lead to some depression. But as in any grieving process, the change in mood should be short-lived; there is resolution and acceptance as time passes. Losses do not make one lose interest in living to one's fullest capacity. It is certainly not normal for an elderly person to be chronically depressed. This is the same type of ageism that once led to the dismissal of dementia as "normal."

Mood Disorders in Children and Adolescents

Although both major depression and bipolar disorder usually first manifest themselves in the young adult years, younger people can suffer from mood disorders as well. As has often happened in psychiatry, the understanding of mood disorders in children was long hampered by misconceptions based on theory rather than on fact. For many years it was believed that children were too psychologically immature to experience true depression. As a more empirical approach to psychiatric problems replaced those rooted in theory, it has become clear that children do indeed get depressed. Complicated classification systems for mood disorders in children have been postulated, trying to separate out children with mood symptoms alone from those also showing many behavioral difficulties in addition to their mood changes. Some even theorize that those with aggressive behavior are different from those with predominately fearful behavior. It's become rather clear that major depression and bipolar disorder as they occur in children are really the same illnesses as in adults and that the same diagnostic criteria apply. Mood disorders seem to be less common in children, especially younger ones, and thus risk for developing them does appear to increase with age.

Major Depression in Children and Adolescents

As I stated above, children do indeed get depressed and often show the same symptoms as adults. Children may be tearful and look quite sad, or they may be irritable or petulant. They can have the same changes in self-attitude as adults do and can feel guilty or responsible for having caused trouble and show the same low self-esteem and self-reproach. Loss of interest in usually pleasurable activities, low energy and fatigue, and poor concentration can also be seen in children. The vegetative signs, of course, are often present: poor sleep, and loss of appetite with weight change. The same uncomfortable bodily sensations that plague adults can lead to complaints of "tummyaches," and headaches are common too.

Children, especially young children, do not have the verbal skills to describe a concept as subtle as mood, and so the changes in behavior caused by their unhappiness and vegetative symptoms can sometimes be the only clue to the onset of a major depressive episode. For example, they may become listless and lose interest in school or play. Children who are depressed may suddenly revert to behaviors they had outgrown. For example, children who have been toilet trained for months or even years will begin to wet themselves again. They may resume sucking their thumbs. Sometimes children who are depressed develop phobias or unwarranted fears; they may suddenly show fear of animals, be afraid of the dark, or refuse to go to school.

Adolescents, of course, get depressed too. Like old age, adolescence is a time of life when symptoms of depression are often explained away as being so common as to be normal. Again, this is simply not the case.

Like young children, depressed adolescents can have a hard time expressing emotional distress verbally, and behavioral changes may be their most prominent symptoms. They may express their uncomfortable feelings through angry, destructive behavior rather than lethargy and listlessness, and sudden aggressiveness in a formerly compliant teenager may signal the onset of depression. This behavior is sometimes said to represent a "depressive equivalent." Adolescents can also show the same symptoms as depressed adults. The boy who loses interest in bodybuilding or the girl who doesn't bother with her hair anymore may be showing the decreased sense of self-worth and even hopelessness that are typical symptoms of affective disorder. I will be discussing drug and alcohol abuse and affective disorder in a later section. Here it is enough to say that the onset of chemical dependency can be a symptom of major depression. I suppose the key word in much of this is "change." Affective disorder is episodic in its course. Any change in activity level, dropping grades, or loss of interest in friends, dating, sports, and so forth may indicate that a change in mood is occurring, and that change may be due to major depression.

Because mood is a concept that adolescents and especially children are to some extent unfamiliar with, they may not complain of feeling depressed, and it often is what others notice about their behavior that signals something is wrong. Because of this, young people with major depression are especially liable to be misdiagnosed. Young children who show a lot of fearfulness may be mislabeled as suffering from a phobia or another anxiety disorder. Those who are listless and uninterested in school may be considered "learning disabled." The worst type of "misdiagnosis," of course, is when they are called "lazy" or "troublemakers" at school or at home. As I stated above, teens may show predominantly behavioral problems and thus be labeled delinquent. Some studies have suggested that many children and adolescents who refuse to attend school are actually depressed.

In the section in chapter 6 called "The Heredity of Mood Disorders," I will discuss a possible link between major depression and the strange eating disorder called anorexia nervosa. In this disorder, which is most common in adolescents, especially girls, patients stop eating, lose a tremendous amount of weight, and may seem intent on starving themselves. Research indicates that some patients who have been called anorexic may instead have major depression, and some treatments for major depression seem to help even in patients with classic anorexia nervosa. As with many links of this sort, further research may shed light on both illnesses.

The medications used to treat major depression in children and adolescents are the same ones used in adults. Imipramine, the first modern antidepressant, has had the most study in the treatment of depression in young people, and the course of treatment is essentially the same as in adults. The doses used are of course lower in younger children, and the treatment dose is often calculated by using body weight: 3–5 milligrams per kilogram is an average range. In adolescents the dose is more comparable to that used in adults.

ECT is rarely used in children, perhaps because the more severe cases of depression that require it are very rare in this age range.

Bipolar Disorder in Children and Adolescents

Bipolar disorder has been documented in children and adolescents. As with major depression, it becomes more common as one looks at older age groups and seems much less prevalent in children than in adults. Some studies indicate that the appearance of manic symptoms at a young age indicates a severe form of the illness with a worse prognosis. These children often have a strong family history of a mood disorder, especially bipolar disorder. As in major depression, the symptoms of the manic state in children are very similar to those seen in adults, but the behavioral changes can be the most prominent.

As you might expect, children with manic or hypomanic moods can look very much like children with "hyperactivity" or, as this problem is now called, attention deficit disorder (ADD). In both problems the child cannot sit still and is extremely talkative, disruptive at school, and always getting into trouble at home. The important differentiating characteristic is the cyclic nature of the change in activity level. ADD children often are shown to have a learning disability when they undergo psychological testing. Also, as I said earlier, young people with bipolar disorder often have a strong family history of mood disorder.

The treatment is the same as for adults; lithium is the mainstay (see "The Treatment of Bipolar Disorder" in chapter 4).

Suicide in Children and Adolescents

Perhaps no other psychiatric problem has received as much attention in the media, in schools, and among mental health professionals in recent years as adolescent suicide. The frightening truth is that self-destructive behavior among young people has truly increased; the suicide rate for persons between the ages of ten and twenty-four has risen more than 200 percent since 1960. Suicide is the third leading cause of death in those under twenty-five; almost one-quarter of all adolescent mortality is due to suicide, and two-thirds of all suicides occur in the twenty to twenty-four-year age group.

In 1987 researchers asked 380 high-school students about suicidal behavior and found that 60 percent had thought about killing themselves and 9 percent had actually made a suicide attempt. Perhaps the most tragic statistic of all is that fewer than half of those in the study who had attempted suicide had received psychiatric treatment of any kind.

The reasons for these frightening numbers are the subject of great debate, which I will not attempt to summarize here. The points I wish to drive home are that suicide is most often seen in persons suffering from a mood disorder; that children and adolescents suffer from mood disorders; and that, *as a group*, adolescents attempt and complete suicide at a significantly higher rate than adults. This means that the adolescent with a mood disorder is doubly at risk and that it is therefore even more vital that mood disorders be recognized and treated in this age group.

Adolescence is a time of many emotional changes, when separation from parents and family and a struggle for emotional autonomy reaches its height. Sexuality issues and sexual feelings may conflict with parental and societal expectations. It is a time when the comforting social structure of high school is about to end and the need for financial self-sufficiency begins. For these reasons late adolescence can strain one's ability to cope to its limit. It is *not*, however, a time when it is "normal" to be depressed or to have suicidal thoughts. The emergence of symptoms of depression should never be brushed off simply because they occur in an adolescent. On the contrary, as the statistics above indicate, in adolescence depressive symptoms should be looked at even more seriously, and measures to get the adolescent evaluated for major depression should be taken without delay.

Review the symptoms of major depression (see chapter 2) and remember that adolescents sometimes "mask" their depression with aggressive, destructive behavior and substance abuse.

Mood Disorders in Women

There are many disputes among the scientists who do research in mood disorders, but almost all agree that major depression is more common among women than among men. Most studies indicate that it is almost twice as common. At one time it was thought that this difference was an invalid finding, that it only *seemed* that more women than men had major depression because women were more willing to come for treatment. Since most studies on affective disorder were conducted in hospitals and university or medical center mental health clinics, such an explanation was difficult to disprove. Because such studies were done on groups of people who had already come for treatment, if women are more willing to come than men, it might appear that more women suffered from major depression if one simply counted the relative numbers of men and women who came to the clinic.

Recent studies on the prevalence of psychiatric problems have attempted to avoid this problem (called ascertainment bias by statisticians) by interviewing representative samples of very large groups of people—whole cities in fact—rather than looking at hospital charts or interviewing patients visiting mental health clinics. People in the community were picked at random and interviewed, and psychiatric diagnoses were made. These studies, designed to be free of ascertainment bias, seem to bear out the older ones and to verify that depression is indeed more common in females than in males. The two-to-one ratio still held. (Bipolar disorder, by the way, is found equally often in males and females.) Is there something different about depression in women that explains this finding?

"Involutional Melancholia"

At one time a certain type of depressive disorder was thought to exist almost exclusively in women. "Involutional melancholia" was considered a unique form of depression, given a separate diagnosis in earlier versions of the *Diagnostic and Statistical Manual* of the American Psychiatric Association. This disorder was at one time linked causally to menopause, but this link is no longer thought to be valid. In addition, as studies on depression accumulated data on the true prevalence of this symdrome, it became clear that "involutional melancholia" was common in men as well as in women, and its identity as a woman's disease dropped away. At that point the concept came to be associated with old age, and it may still have some usefulness as a clinical picture common to depression in older people (see "Major Depression in the Elderly" above).

Postpartum Depression

Postpartum depression, however, is a very real condition seen exclusively in females. "Postpartum" refers to the time after giving birth, and mood problems during this period are extremely common. For many years, all kinds of psychiatric problems were described in women who had recently given birth. Most of these "psychiatric" problems were actually periods of disorientation and delirium that probably had medical causes such as dehydration, blood loss, infections, and other problems that have largely disappeared with modern obstetrical techniques. Nevertheless, mood changes do occur in the postpartum period that do not seem to have anything to do with the trauma of labor and delivery.

The range of symptom types is wide, and the range of severity is even wider. In one study, over 90 percent of the women interviewed reported crying spells they could not explain, perhaps the mildest form of the disorder. A smaller number report mood changes that are persistent and cause some disturbance in their functioning, and a very small percentage have serious, debilitating mood changes that may last months.

Immediately after the baby is born there is often a period of euphoria—a very good mood. The depression usually occurs two to five days after the birth. The depression may be limited to brief crying spells, or the full major depressive syndrome may appear. The guilty qualities of the mood change may be prominent; often this takes the form of concerns about the baby's health. ("The baby cries too much; I must have done something wrong during my pregnancy; I didn't take good care of myself.") Women sometimes feel they don't love the baby enough. They may feel some resentment at the prospect of so many new responsibilities, and so they question their commitment and love. ("I should enjoy changing diapers; if I don't that must mean I'm going to be a bad mother.")

The biological factors that have been implicated in this problem are, as you might suspect, hormonal. During pregnancy, the body produces high levels of various hormones to maintain the blood supply of the uterus and support the baby developing inside. These are the "female" steroids. During the delivery of the baby there is significant pain, blood loss, and other physical stress, and then the "stress" steroids such as cortisol are produced. Some have speculated that the euphoria seen immediately after birth is caused by the high levels of these steroids, and that when these levels drop a "steroid withdrawal" causes the mood change. It may be that in most women this change is quickly compensated for as the body recovers from pregnancy and birth, and so "the baby blues" are mild and transient. In some women, however, the hormonal changes may precipitate a chain of events that produces the change in brain chemistry causing the symptoms of major depression. Whether women who have the more severe forms of postpartum depression are at risk for later spontaneous episodes of mood disorder is not known for certain.

Premenstrual Mood Disorders

Any poorly understood medical problem that receives a great deal of publicity in the general media can strike terror into the heart of a practicing physician who is called on to diagnose it, treat it, or even comment on it. People easily assume that anything they hear on television is true and forget that selling soap is more important to television producers than are medical facts. So it's with some trepidation that I will discuss what is popularly known as premenstrual syndrome (PMS). Despite the two-page magazine articles written by people with (perhaps) a degree in journalism that purport to tell you all about the psychological symptoms caused by menstruation, a recent paper in the *American Journal of Psychiatry* stated that "despite 50 years of study, relatively little is known about the relationship of menstruation and mood disorders."* Nevertheless, there are some facts that most experts agree on, and enough attention has been paid to this problem that it certainly bears discussion in a book on mood disorders.

It is quite clear that many women experience a variety of physical and emotional symptoms starting about five days before the onset of menstruation and continuing for about two days after their menstrual flow starts. Those who do not have these symptoms during the rest of the month have been said to have premenstrual syndrome.

Exactly what the symptoms of premenstrual syndrome are is perhaps the most difficult aspect of the controversy surrounding this problem. Studies that have set out to define the syndrome vary greatly depending on the research interest of the investigator. Psychologists and psychiatrists have tended to study emotional symptoms, and gynecologists have focused on physical ones. Endocrinologists have concentrated on hormone levels. All claim to be

*D. R. Rubinow, et al., "Premenstrual syndromes: Overview from a methodological perspective," in *American Journal of Psychiatry* 141 (1984): 163-72.

looking at women with "PMS," but whether they are studying the same or different groups of patients is unknown. Some studies did not differentiate between symptoms occurring only during the premenstrual period and symptoms that were present most of the month but got worse premenstrually. The common symptoms that usually are considered to represent PMS are mood changes, including depression or irritability, and several physical symptoms including water retention and consequent weight gain, appetite disturbance (often an increase in appetite with "carbohydrate craving"), sleep changes (usually insomnia), and tiredness and impaired concentration. Many other symptoms have in one study or another been thought to be part of the syndrome; a total of 150 symptoms have been considered to vary with the menstrual cycle! The result of this confusion has been an explosion of women noticing one or another of these 150 symptoms during the premenstrual period for several months and then diagnosing themselves as having PMS.

The crucial question in investigating this problem is this: Is there a discrete group of women who share certain symptoms during the premenstrual period and not at other times? There are enough reasonably well-designed studies suggesting a tentative yes to this question that the American Psychiatric Association debated adding PMS as a diagnostic category. This step sparked a tremendous controversy, mainly because many felt that adding a category for a condition seen exclusively in women was stigmatizing and sexist, especially if what was being called PMS (or as DSM-III-R wanted to label it, "late luteal phase dysphoric disorder") was simply a variant of affective disorder.

Just as "involutional melancholia" was thrown out as a diagnostic category because it was affective disorder given another name when it occurred in older people, so was this proposed diagnosis. It doesn't make sense to call affective disorder something different when it occurs in women and gets worse (as it seems a lot of problems get worse) during the premenstrual period.

What sort of studies led the American Psychiatric Association to propose this diagnosis? In one,* several hundred women were asked to rate their mood on a scale from zero (not at all depressed) to 100 (very depressed) every day for several months. The results

*D. R. Rubinow, et al., "Prospective assessment of menstrually related mood disorders," in *American Journal of Psychiatry* 141 (1984): 684–86.

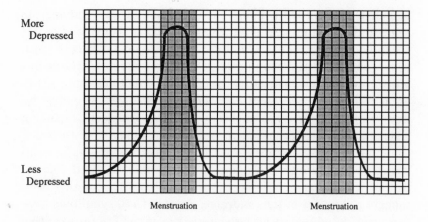

Figure 4   Depression levels across the menstrual cycle.

were graphed out, and of the first twenty women in the study, eight (40 percent) had graphs that looked something like figure 4. This is a striking and clear-cut indication that some women do indeed have significant mood changes during the premenstrual period. Is this affective disorder or PMS? I think most experts would concur that there is not enough agreement on what PMS is to answer this question. Another fact may point the way toward an answer, though. In studies where women with major depression were asked about their mood changes during the premenstrual period, a high percentage said they had significant premenstrual depression, often several times that of women without affective disorder. Women with affective disorder thus may have a worsening of symptoms during the premenstrual period. What are the symptoms these women report? Low mood, irritability, desire to avoid others, guilty thoughts—in short, the typical symptoms of major depression. There are reported cases of suicidal behavior as well.

The menstrual cycle is characterized by the rhythmic rise and fall of several hormones, primarily estrogen and progesterone, the "female" sex steroids. Do women with premenstrual exacerbation of mood disorders have some hormonal imbalance? Again, we lack good studies. Some studies of women said to have PMS (which may or may not include those with premenstrual exacerbation of affective disorder) have shown an abnormal ratio of progesterone to estrogen in symptomatic patients. Others have not found this characteristic. Attempts to treat premenstrual symptoms (psychological and physical) by manipulating hormone levels have been uniformly disappointing. If there is such a disorder as PMS, there is not much to be gained by diagnosing it at this point, since there is no effective treatment. This does not mean, however, that none of the symptoms associated with the premenstrual period can be treated. On the contrary, many can, and the emotional symptoms may be some of the most effectively treated.

So what is the relation of premenstrual mood symptoms to affective disorder? We do not know, but it seems to me that one way to make sense out of the available facts is to borrow the formulation I presented concerning postpartum depression. The hormonal changes of menstruation are so powerful that they cause minor mood changes in many, perhaps even most, women. One is almost tempted to call this "normal." In some women, however, the mood changes are severe. Many women with severe premenstrual mood changes have had episodes of major depression. It may be that, as with postpartum depression, in women with a predisposition for affective disorder, the hormonal changes set off a change in neurotransmitters that causes symptoms of major depression.

One very practical conclusion to be drawn from this confusing set of facts is that some women who have mood problems premenstrually may in fact suffer from affective disorder, specifically major depression, and may get relief when treated with antidepressants. Some women may have mild symptoms of depression all the time that they ignore, learn to live with, or consider normal. When their mood gets much worse during the premenstrual period, however, it may interfere with their functioning. This group may label themselves as having PMS and see a gynecologist. If the gynecologist is adept enough to diagnose a mood disorder and suggest antidepressant medication or refer them to a psychiatrist, they may get relief. If not, they may undergo expensive hormone studies and be tried on vitamins, hormone replacement, and other ineffective medications.

Premenstrual mood variation in patients who are being treated for major depression can cause an episodic worsening of symptoms that is confusing to both patient and doctor. Another case study will illustrate this problem.

Mary was successfully treated for a major depressive episode, but her premenstrual exacerbation of depression caused a lot of confusion. When she first came to my office Mary's symptoms were severe. They had started abruptly after a few nights of sleeplessness, and in Mary they took the form of severe anxiety, fearfulness, and even dread. Her powerful feelings of impending catastrophe made her desperate and were severe enough to cause her to be suicidal, so that she was admitted to the hospital. I immediately started Mary on imipramine, and because she was so upset I added a small dose of antipsychotic medication.

The first confusing event was the almost complete resolution of her severe symptoms after only two days of taking imipramine. Some patients do get symptom relief from antidepressants in significantly less than the more usual two to four weeks, but this was extraordinary. Mary went home after only a few more days and came back for a follow-up appointment the next week. When I saw her she was looking so much better and was in such good spirits that I completely stopped her antipsychotic medication.

About ten days later I got a call from Mary's husband, who said she was sleepless again and had started to become fearful and "paranoid." Since the only change had been discontinuing the antipsychotic, I told her to start taking it again. The medication helped Mary get to sleep, and in a day or two she was much better again.

Mary and her husband were glad the antipsychotic was helping, but I was worried—perhaps Mary didn't have affective disorder but had schizophrenia instead. That might account for her rapid recovery in the hospital and her sudden deterioration after the antipsychotic medication was stopped.

I saw Mary the next week, and she again seemed to be doing extremely well. I questioned her closely about her symptoms, looking for any hint of the type of bizarre mind-control experiences and hallucinations of schizophrenia. There were none. Her symptoms seemed limited to a change in mood; in fact, by this time Mary was comfortable enough talking to me that she admitted that her fearfulness and "paranoia" had come from her thoughts that she was a bad person and that someone was going to find out and hurt her. This was sounding *more* like affective disorder, not less. But how could I account for the unusual pattern of symptoms? I told her to keep taking the antipsychotic medication for now.

I saw Mary several more times and tapered off her antipsychotic level a little. For no particular reason, I had Mary get a blood test for the antidepressant level.

At the next appointment Mary said, "You know, I still get those fearful thoughts and sleepless nights every once in a while. But I just take a few extra tranquilizers and I'm OK. I've noticed that it's always right before my period. Do you think I have PMS?"

As Mary was saying this, I picked up the lab slip with her antidepressant level from my desk. Her level was in the therapeutic range, but just barely so. "Do you remember if you were about to get your period when you first got sick, before you were admitted to the hospital?" I asked. "Yes," she replied. "In fact, I think it started the day after I was admitted."

I asked a few more questions, and the pattern emerged. Mary did indeed have major depression, but her mood was strikingly affected by the hormonal changes in the premenstrual period. Her sudden "recovery" in the hospital was probably a spontaneous improvement related to coming out of the premenstrual hormonal state. Her abrupt "relapse" was not caused by discontinuing the antipsychotic but was a premenstrual exacerbation of her major depression. She was taking enough antidepressant to get good symptom control during most of the monthly cycle, but the added stress of the premenstrual changes "overpowered" the effects of the medication and caused a breakthrough of symptoms. The barely therapeutic lab result supported this reasoning. We raised the dose of antidepressant to get her more solidly into the therapeutic range, and her symptoms were completely controlled.

This section has included two important facts about major depression in women: the disorder occurs as frequently in women as in men, and the symptoms of major depression seem to be precipitated or exacerbated in women during times of dramatic hormonal changes—the premenstrual period, the postpartum period, and possibly the menopausal period. The conclusion seems almost inevitable that there must be some link between the female hormonal system and the neurochemistry of major depression. What this link is remains a mystery. Perhaps being female is necessary for the expression of certain genes for affective disorder (as being male is necessary for the expression of some forms of baldness) and a particular hormonal state that only women can have confers an added vulnerability to major depression.

I'll editorialize a bit here. It *does* seem sexist to me to call affective disorder something different in women just because they are more liable than men to develop it. Men are more likely to develop high blood pressure, yet there's no such thing as "masculine hypertension!"

Depression and Stroke

Few medical problems appear as suddenly or cause such devastating impairment as cerebrovascular accident. The common name for this problem, stroke, is derived from these qualities, since the victim is often "struck down" as if by a bolt of lightning going from health and normal functioning to paralysis and often unconsciousness in minutes or even seconds. A stroke occurs when the blood supply to part of the brain is suddenly cut off. This can occur for a number of reasons, but the most common is blockage in a blood vessel, usually a blood clot caused by the same kind of circulatory disease—atherosclerosis—that causes heart attack. The brain cannot function for even a short time without the oxygen blood carries to it, and the part of the brain affected immediately ceases to work. If the blood supply is not restored in a very few minutes, brain cells die.

The symptoms of stroke vary with the size of the blood vessel affected. If a tiny branch vessel is blocked, the symptoms may be minor; if one of the major vessels is blocked, there can be paralysis of an entire side of the body. Depending on which part of the brain is affected, speech is often impaired, either because the brain area coordinating the muscles of speech is damaged or because the language area of the brain is affected.

It seems no wonder that patients who have had a stroke become depressed. Within minutes one can change from a well-coordinated athlete or musician into a profoundly handicapped invalid—speech slurred, one arm hanging useless, dragging leg and foot in a shuffle.

For many years the high frequency of depression in stroke patients was dismissed as understandable in light of their impairment. As psychiatry became more interested in the diagnosis of affective disorder, however, some interesting facts were noted. Most striking was that a much larger number of stroke patients than expected seemed to develop not the expected reactive or psychological form of depression, but the full-blown major depressive syndrome. Some seemed to experience a major depressive episode simultaneously with the other stroke symptoms; in a sense, they seemed to be depressed as soon as they regained consciousness. Also, these depressed patients got better with the usual treatments for major depression, antidepressant medication and ECT. Moreover, if they did not receive medical treatment for depression, their mood symptoms lasted six months to a year, just the time a major depressive episode would be expected to last. When a group of patients who had had strokes were compared with a group of patients with equally disabling injuries that did not involve the brain, the stroke patients were found to be more frequently and more severely depressed. When the psychiatric symptoms of severely depressed stroke patients were compared with those of patients with major depression in a psychiatric hospital, the types of symptoms were almost identical. Further studies have shown that nearly half of patients who have strokes develop symptoms of major depression within two years.

The almost inevitable conclusion is that when the brain is injured in a cerebrovascular accident, the same process is often set in motion that causes the symptoms of major depression. The symptoms, the time course of the untreated illness, and the response to treatment are identical. In effect, the stroke produces the syndrome of major depression in every way, presumably in patients who would not otherwise show such symptoms.

These findings have tremendous importance for stroke patients, their families, and their physicians. When a person who has had a stroke becomes depressed, it is imperative that the diagnosis of poststroke major depressive syndrome be considered and that the patient be treated appropriately. Many of the impairments caused by stroke—muscle weakness and loss of coordination, for example—need to be treated with physical therapy and sometimes more specialized rehabilitation such as speech therapy. These treatments require tremendous motivation and commitment from the patient. Patients who are depressed will not have the emotional resources necessary to participate in their rehabilitation—may in fact feel so hopeless that they do not believe any recovery of function is possible and so refuse rehabilitation therapy. They may simply want to lie in bed; yet if this is allowed, already weakened muscles can waste away, and sometimes severe muscle and joint degeneration called contracture can develop that makes physical therapy painful and more difficult. The lethargic, bedridden, partially paralyzed person is prone to chronic medical problems such as bedsores, and even life-threatening medical problems can supervene—pneumonia and phlebitis, for example. (Phlebitis is the formation of a blood clot in an inflamed vein, usually the large veins of the legs. Such clots can break loose and travel through the blood vessels to the brain, causing another stroke, or sometimes to the lungs, causing an often fatal cardiovascular collapse known as pulmonary embolism.)

Stroke victims who are showing symptoms of depression should not be dismissed as simply discouraged at their new infirmity or demoralized at their loss of health. Major depression may occur in as many as 50 percent of stroke patients. What a tragedy if the mood symptoms are ignored or considered untreatable and the patient dies from complications of inactivity! Just as the symptoms of major depression are often dismissed as "normal" in the elderly and in adolescents, it is not difficult to explain away depression in a stroke patient. An appropriate course of treatment, however, either with antidepressant medication or with ECT, can speed recovery from the physical impairments by restoring a normal mood state so that the patient can participate in the rehabilitative treatments necessary for recovery.

Aside from the clinical implications discussed above, the recognition that stroke can cause major depression has had major significance for neuroscientists interested in the biological basis of mood disorders. Much of what we know about the nervous system was discovered by studying people who had suffered brain damage from strokes as well as other illnesses and injuries. By carefully cataloging the pattern of symptoms and signs seen following an injury and then carefully observing the exact location and extent of damage to the brain after the victim's eventual death, it was possible to "map out" many areas of the brain and their functions. The most elementary discovery was that the muscles on one side of the body are controlled by the opposite side of the brain. For example, a blood vessel blockage that damages the left side of the brain will cause paralysis on the right side of the body. By correlating the site of injury in the brain with the operation disrupted when that injury occurs, many brain functions have been localized. Most muscle movements, bodily sensations, vision, hearing, and even more complicated activities such as some language operations have been found to have well-defined locations. With the development of sophisticated imaging techniques such as CAT (computerized axial tomography) and now MRI (magnetic resonance imaging), the procedures known as "brain scans," damaged areas of the brain can be mapped in living patients in a painless, noninvasive way, without the need to wait for postmortem examination. These techniques have tremendously aided this method of clinical research and accelerated the acquisition of knowledge about the organization of the brain.

Has the study of stroke patients with depression allowed localization of a "mood center" in the brain? Not quite yet, but there have been some intriguing findings that hint at the existence of such a center. First, patients who have had strokes involving the left side of the brain develop depression more frequently and are more severely depressed than patients who have "right-sided" strokes. Second, the closer to the front of the left side of the brain the damage is, the more severe the depression.

Animal experiments have shown that damage near the front of the brain on one side only will produce a widespread depletion of neurotransmitters in the brain. A single damaged area seems to affect the balance of neurotransmitters throughout many brain areas.

Cutting a power line as it enters an office building will make all the lights in the building go out, whereas cutting a smaller cable inside may knock out only the lights on one floor. Similarly, there seems to be a "cable" of nerve fibers that passes through the front of the brain on one side and then fans out, traveling to many areas of the brain. Such a system might be responsible for setting a tone or level of chemical activity necessary for efficient brain functioning. It may be that when one of the main structures of this system is disrupted, a whole spectrum of brain activity is also disrupted—sleep, appetite, energy level, concentration, ability to experience pleasure—in short the whole collection of experiences psychiatrists have grouped together and called mood.

A manic episode following brain injury is a much rarer event, the incidence being a small fraction of that of poststroke depression. Nevertheless, a recent study has shown that patients who develop manic symptoms following brain injury often show damage to the right side of the surface of the brain and to some particular deeper structures. Many of those studied had a family history of mood disorder or had themselves had an episode of major depression or mania. The findings are therefore more difficult to interpret, but they suggest that right-sided brain structures may also be involved in regulating mood.

The investigation of poststroke depression has been an extremely fertile field in neuropsychiatry. It has pointed toward a localization of the brain system that may be involved in major depression. Once this is established, we will be one giant step closer to discovering the cause of major depression and other mood disorders.

Depression and Pain

Like the symptom of depression, pain is a universal human experience. As we have seen, depression the symptom can sometimes widen and deepen to include a whole collection of other symptoms that severely impair the sufferer and form a "syndrome" that takes on a life of its own and needs specific medical treatment. The same seems to be true for pain, and the term *chronic pain syndrome* describes a comparable collection of pain-related symptoms.

Chronic low-back pain is the commonest such syndrome, and chronic pelvic pain, especially in women, is also frequent. Chronic headache is a widespread problem as well.

It's difficult to define a chronic pain syndrome with precision. Victims complain of chronic—meaning long-standing and constant—pain that is poorly explained by medical findings and seems to interfere with normal functioning out of proportion to them.

Notice I said *poorly* explained and interfering *out of proportion* to the findings. Chronic pain syndrome does not refer to pain that seems to be totally psychological; usually these patients have real medical problems or pathology—for example, arthritis in the lumbar (lower back) or cervical (neck) spine or a history of pelvic infections or surgery that can cause chronic discomfort. What distinguishes them is that their complaints of pain and the handicapping effects of their pain are much greater than in other patients who seem to have the same medical histories and the same amount of pathology. They request more pain medication, they refuse to attend to jobs or housework, and they may complain that their pain prevents them from sleeping properly. They lose interest in sex, and lose weight. They are irritable and can't enjoy anything. These patients were thought to have more severe symptoms for a variety of reasons. The vague concept of low pain threshold was invoked. They were thought to suffer from personality problems; perhaps they were "addictive personalities" and were exaggerating symptoms to get narcotics from their doctors. They were sometimes thought to be malingering, hoping for disability insurance payments. All too often they were simply called "crocks" and ignored. I hope that by now, however, this collection of symptoms seems very familiar to you; it includes many of the same ones that together characterize major depression. About fifteen years ago, special hospital units were beginning to be set up for patients, usually addicted to pain medications such as narcotics, who had debilitating pain not well explained by medical findings. The treatment teams of the best units included medical doctors, surgeons (often neurosurgeons, who most often do back operations), anesthesiologists (who in effect are the specialists in pain relief), and also psychiatrists. The psychiatrists noticed that many of the pain patients had all the symptoms of major depression. In studying this group further, they noted that their family histories included a higher-than-expected prevalence of alcohol problems and depression. (Further discussion of the relation of alcohol abuse to mood disorders and the genetics of mood disorders will be found in the next chapter.) As you might expect, trials of antidepressant medications on these patients sometimes produced dramatic results; not only did the symptoms of depression get better, but the pain was relieved as well.

It has become apparent that there is a close relation between chronic pain syndrome and depression. One study* that attempted to define this relationship more clearly gave dexamethasone suppression tests to a group of patients with chronic pain who had been referred to a pain treatment center (see the section "Tests for Affective Disorder" in chapter 3). Some of the patients who had symptoms of major depression did indeed have positive test results, and pain patients who did not meet the criteria for major depression had uniformly negative tests. This seems to indicate that chronic pain and major depression are two distinct problems that can indeed be separated out. But this clarity becomes clouded again when one considers another fact: antidepressants can give significant pain relief to patients who are impaired by their pain but do not seem depressed. The doses required for pain relief in "nondepressed" chronic pain sufferers are usually lower than those used to treat depression.

Because the relationship is not well defined by available clinical facts and theory, the concept of the chronic pain syndrome is said to have become "enmeshed" with that of depression. This characterization perhaps emphasizes what we don't know rather than what we do understand about depression and pain.

We do understand, for example, that pain can be a symptom of major depression. Headaches and vague abdominal pains are common, but other types of pain are seen as well—indeed, as many kinds of pain as there are body parts and organs. In some people who have major depression, pain is prominent; in fact, they may attribute their other symptoms—weight loss, insomnia, and so forth—to the pain. They may even attribute their depressed mood to their pain, and this can lead to problems, especially if their doctor is "a guy with a hammer." Perhaps you've heard the old saying, "If you're a guy with a hammer, everything looks like a nail." It's possible for some doctors, particularly specialists, to focus only on their specialty and to miss a more general problem such as depression. I have seen many patients said to have "irritable bowel syndrome" (gastroenterologists), "migraine" or "cluster headaches" (neurologists), fibromyositis (rheumatologists), and other assorted maladies who were actually suffering from major depression.

*R. D. France, et al., "Differentiation of depression from chronic pain with the dexamethasone depression test and the DSM-III," in *American Journal of Psychiatry* 141 (1984): 1577–97.

Often, though, the depressed person with prominent pain symptoms is the one missing the broader picture, not the doctor. I've known of patients who have gotten very angry, even stormed out of the office, when their medical doctor suggested a psychiatric consultation. Several times a year I'll get a phone call from one of my medical colleagues with an "emergency" patient with headaches or some other pain symptom who has seen doctor after doctor without receiving relief of the pain or an explanation of its source and who is now "very depressed and desperate." I promise to see the person the very same day, after usual office hours if necessary, only to get a phone call later canceling the appointment. The idea of seeing a psychiatrist is just too threatening for some people.

I think several factors conspire to effect such a doubly unhappy outcome. The first is the Cartesian dichotomy that basically divides all human experiences into those of the mind and those of the body and states that the two "realms" do not affect one another. The hypothetical wall dividing these realms has been crumbling stone by stone, but it is still a high one. The term coined to express the relationship, *psychosomatic*, has come to be almost pejorative, implying that "It's all in your head." We have come to accept that chronic tension can worsen peptic ulcers and that "type A personalities" may have early heart attacks (though this last has become doubtful), but for many people the idea that depression can cause pain and that psychiatrists are the depression experts in the medical community is still so foreign that it prevents them from getting the treatment they need. The second and perhaps more important factor is the stigma associated with "mental illness." This is so important that I will discuss it in some detail in a later section (see "Stigma" in chapter 7).

Another clearly understood fact about pain and depression is that pain from existing medical problems can be exacerbated by depression. Symptoms of arthritis, back problems, and some of the painful complications of chronic medical conditions such as the nerve pain called neuropathy seen in diabetes can get much worse. Pain that was being adequately controlled with medication no longer responds. This problem is especially difficult to diagnose correctly, since both doctor and patient can easily assume that the original problem is worsening when in fact a second problem—depression—has arisen.

The last fact about pain is one I mentioned earlier: antidepressant medications sometimes alleviate pain symptoms in people who do not seem very depressed. This fact has been the most difficult to explain. Since the antidepressants that help most affect the neurotransmitter serotonin (the drugs amitriptyline and trazodone) it has been suggested the patients who develop chronic pain may have some imbalance of the serotonin system that these antidepressants correct—that the problem has nothing to do with affective disorder but is relieved by a "side effect" of some antidepressants. Others have theorized that this pain is an "equivalent" of depression—depression in another form.

Over the years, I have tried many ways to explain to my patients the associations and connections between physical symptoms and psychiatric symptoms. Some have enough medical sophistication to discuss such things as the autonomic nervous system, adrenaline surges, and so forth. But there's a rather simple-minded statement that vividly sums up these complicated theoretical problems: "The brain *is* connected to the rest of the body, you know!" As medical scientists grow more familiar with the complexities of the body, the connections become more and more evident. One discovery is that many substances once thought to be exclusively related to "the body" have functions in the brain as well. Cholecystokinin is secreted by the gastrointestinal tract and helps regulate how fast the stomach empties food into the intestine. Recently it was discovered that cholecystokinin is also a neurotransmitter! It is found in brain cells, and receptors for it are found in the brain as well. It may be involved in the sensations of hunger and satiety. Receptors for testosterone, the male sex hormone secreted by the testes, have also been found in the brain, though their function, as well as the role of testosterone in sexual behavior, is sketchy at this point.

One of the first breakthroughs, and perhaps the most startling, linking the experience of pain with the chemistry of the brain was the discovery of opiate receptors in certain areas of the nervous system. An opiate is a substance derived from the opium poppy, and various related drugs manufactured from this plant are collectively referred to as narcotics (from the Greek *narkotikos*, "benumbing"). Opiate or narcotic compounds include opium, morphine, codeine, heroin, and many others. The valuable medical use of these substances is their analgesic (pain-relieving) quality; they also can produce a state of euphoria, and it is this effect that accounts for their widespread abuse. (I'll return to this point about euphoria later.) Opiates were of course well known for centuries before the discovery of neurotransmitters, but as pharmaceutical researchers worked to produce safer and more effective pain medications from opium, they discovered new substances with some interesting properties indicating that opiates might mimic a chemical produced by the brain that is involved in the experience of pain. They found that a slight alteration in the chemical structure of an effective analgesic could cause it to block the effect of other narcotics (accounting for the name of these compounds: narcotic antagonists). This result would make sense only if there were receptors for opiates in the nervous system. If such a receptor worked like other known neurotransmitter receptors, a chemical that mimicked the neurotransmitter very closely in structure would also mimic its function (like a copy of a latchkey good enough to open a lock). Another substance that is close but not an exact match in chemical structure might block the original drug's effects (like a key copy that fits into the keyhole but won't turn, yet prevents the door from being opened even by a key that fits).

As neuroscientific techniques became more advanced, the receptors were found in various parts of the brain and spinal cord. Why were they there? Why should the brain have receptors for poppy compounds? The answer, of course, is that the poppy compounds mimic some substance naturally produced in the brain that is involved in the perception of pain. Some of these substances have been isolated from brain preparations and have been called endorphins (from *endo-*, within, and morphine).

An interesting point about the opiate receptors of the nervous system is that they are found not only in brain and spinal cord areas that are known to transmit pain impulses, but in other areas of the brain as well. Some of these other brain areas are in the limbic system, which is poorly understood but seems to be intimately involved in the experience of mood.

Knowledge of narcotic drugs and opiate receptors has thus revealed another one of what must be many direct connections between major depression and chronic pain. Narcotics cause euphoria—definitely a mood change—and there are opiate receptors in the limbic system of the brain, which seems to be involved in mood and mood disorders.

Throughout this book I have emphasized again and again that psychological symptoms, symptoms that affect mental processes and experiences such as abnormal changes in mood can be caused by changes in the *biological* functioning of the body and require medical treatment. In this chapter I have explained that a causal relationship extends in the opposite direction as well. Depression, a condition primarily affecting the mental experience of mood, can cause and exacerbate pain, and not only can psychiatric treatment play an important role in pain relief, but in some cases proper psychiatric treatment can provide almost complete relief of chronic pain.

Seasonal Affective Disorder

In every culture and religion, for as long as humans have recorded their rituals and religious observances, there have been celebrations and rites to mark the end of the short days of winter and the beginning of spring. The Roman Saturnalia, Christmas, Hanukkah, and other holidays cluster around the winter solstice, 22 December, the shortest day of the year. Some ancient civilizations built monumental astronomical observatories to calculate solar eclipses and the biannual solstices and equinoxes. The darkening of the sun seen during an eclipse caused terror and great apprehension among these peoples, and the solstice marking the sun's return was calculated and celebrated by structures such as Stonehenge, the temple of the pharaoh Ramses at Abu-Simbel, and the pyramid observatories of the Incas and Aztecs.

Many species of animals are driven by powerful inner forces attuned to the changes of the seasons, which bring about changes in behavior. Seasonally determined migration of birds and sea mammals and hibernation in bears and other land mammals are so familiar that they no longer elicit the same wonder. But some of the workings and facts of chronobiology (*chronos*, "time") have recently become the topic of newspaper and popular magazine articles with the description of seasonal affective disorder and the use of therapeutic light to treat this fascinating mood disorder.

A recurring theme in the discussion of affective disorder that is scattered through this book is chronobiology, by which I mean the study of how biological events relate to astronomical events. We have talked about how symptoms of mood disorders relate to the twenty-four-hour cycle of the earth's rotation on its axis or, more simply put, the day/night cycle. Early-morning awakening and diurnal mood variation are symptoms of major depression. I made reference in chapter 3 to the circadian rhythm of cortisol secretion by the adrenal glands and to the disruption of this daily cycle in some cases of major depression. In the next chapter I'll discuss how manipulating the sleep cycle affects mood and affective disorder. Earlier in this chapter I discussed the relation between affective disorder and the monthly (lunar?) menstrual cycle. Perhaps it is not surprising that there is also a relation between affective disorder and the twelve-month cycle, the annual cycle of the seasons.

As with many other mood abnormalities, seasonal variation in mood in some persons was noted over and over in the psychiatric research literature before being recognized as a variant of affective disorder. In one of the first textbooks of modern psychiatry, the groundbreaking *Manic-Depressive Illness and Paranoia* by the great German psychiatrist Emil Kraepelin, such a variation is described. The increase of depressive symptoms in the winter months has practically become folklore; the "winter blues" and the "February blahs" are commonly accepted concepts.

Only in the past five years or so, however, has it been recognized through careful, systematic study that some people with affective disorder get depressed in the fall and winter and have normal moods (or sometimes periods of hypomania) in the spring and summer. Because of the seasonal cycle of the illness, it is called seasonal affective disorder (SAD).

Let me make it clear that the depression of SAD is a major depressive episode in all clinical respects: sustained lowering of mood, changes in appetite and sleep, feelings of guilt and self-blame, hopelessness—in short, the whole syndrome. A patient is defined as suffering from SAD when for at least two consecutive years, and for at least three years all together, there has been a regular relation between the onset of the abnormal change in mood and a particular time of year. The most common form of the illness is depression in winter and normal mood (often with brief periods of elation of

hypomania) in summer, but the reverse pattern has also been described—depression in summer and normal mood (or hypomania)
in winter.

Although the depression of SAD meets all the diagnostic criteria for major depression, several mood symptoms seem to be more
common in SAD. As in major depression of any type, people with
SAD have changes in appetite and sleep patterns. The SAD patient,
however, almost always has an *increase* in sleep; complaints of
chronic winter fatigue are very common. Also, an increase in appetite
rather than a decrease is more usual, and SAD patients often gain
weight every winter. Almost two-thirds of patients with SAD report
craving sweets and other carbohydrates. Seasonal depressions seem
generally to be less severe than many episodes of major depression.
Of the large number of SAD patients studied by the original researchers at the National Institute of Mental Health (NIMH), only
1 percent ever needed ECT. Although there do not seem to be many
cases of bipolar disorder with full-blown manic states that show
seasonal variation, most people with SAD have brief periods of elation or hypomania in the summer; this would put them into the
category of bipolar II, further delineating SAD from other variations of affective disorder.

Besides the remarkable seasonal rhythm of SAD, the treatment
of the disorder is truly amazing. The most effective treatment for
SAD is light! Instead of medication, ECT, or other traditional psychiatric interventions, SAD patients sit in front of bright lights for
several hours a day to get better.

This novel treatment was based on the observation that those
who regularly got depressed in the winter would see their depressions lift within days if they traveled south—especially far south,
near the equator. Patients who lived in different parts of the world,
specifically at different latitudes, had winter depressions that were
longer and more severe the farther from the equator they lived. How
could this variation be explained? In these days of air conditioning
and central heating it seemed unlikely that temperature changes
could account for it, so research psychiatrists began to investigate
another factor: light.

Alaska's long winter nights and summer days are familiar to
most Americans from elementary-school geography. Near the poles
of the earth, the seasonal variation in length of daylight is most

pronounced. At the geographical poles, there is literally almost six months of darkness in winter; as one moves south, the hours of daylight on a particular winter day increase. At the equator seasonal variation in daylight hours is minimal, and the days are longer all year round. Once the connection between mood and light was recognized in some patients, it became clear that any change in the duration of their exposure to light could bring about changes in mood. A prolonged period of cloudiness or a change in light intensity at work could also trigger a deterioration in mood in some people.

In 1982 NIMH researchers published a paper in the *American Journal of Psychiatry*, "Bright Artificial Light Treatment of a Manic-Depressive Patient with a Seasonal Mood Cycle." It described how exposing a depressed patient to bright light (about ten times the brightness of ordinary room light) alleviated symptoms of depression. *Every subsequent clinical study has replicated these findings*, a consistency almost unheard of in clinical research. The new variation of affective disorder was included in the diagnostic manual of the American Psychiatric Association in the next revision, less than five years after it was first described—another unheard-of event that reflects the solidity of the evidence and the unequivocal results of well planned and executed research.

Flower growers regularly manipulate the length of daylight and nighttime darkness to produce desired biological events. Anyone who puts a poinsettia plant or a Christmas catcus in a dark closet each evening in the fall to coax it into bloom for the holiday season is performing just such a manipulation. Many other species of plants flower only in response to very precise proportions of light hours and dark hours (called a photoperiod).

Biologists discovered years ago that the seasonally determined variations of animal behaviors such as migration and hibernation were also determined not by temperature changes, but by photoperiod. Once this was discovered, the search was on for a hormone or other substance that was triggered by changes in photoperiod. Soon it was discovered that the secretion of melatonin, a hormone produced by the pineal gland, was strongly influenced by photoperiod. The function of the pineal gland, a cone-shaped body about the size of grape seed buried deep in the convolutions of the brain, had for many years been a mystery. Centuries ago it was thought that perhaps this gland was the seat of the soul. This concept fell into disfavor rather early in the history of scientific medicine, yet no function was found for this organ until 1917, when it was discovered that preparations made from the pineal body of the cow caused changes in pigmentation in tadpoles. In 1958 the chemical (hormone) that caused these changes was isolated and called melatonin, from *Melanin*, the name of the dark skin pigment found in many animals including man. The pineal gland secretes this pigment-regulating hormone, but its function remained obscure and little more than a curiosity. It was even postulated that the pineal body was a vestigial third eye. Some thought that the secretion of melatonin in humans was an evolutionary holdover; animals like the Arctic hare, which changes its color from earthy brown to snow white from season to season had an adaptive use for such a regulatory mechanism, but no such phenomenon could be observed in humans.

Evidence has accumulated over the years, however, suggesting that the pineal body, though perhaps not the seat of the human soul, may be the seat of our internal clock. Through a complicated series of neural connections, the pineal gland receives input from the eyes, and its secretion of melatonin cycles over a twenty-four-hour period, being up at night and down during the day (see fig. 5). Manipulating the light/dark cycle in the research laboratory can affect this cycle as does seasonal variation of photoperiod.

As we trace the connections of the pineal body to other parts of the brain and nervous system, we encounter some very interesting relationships. In addition to the connections to the eyes, the pineal body is known to have connections to the adrenal glands, which secrete cortisol in a diurnal pattern. (Remember that this pattern is disrupted in depression; see, in chapter 3, "Tests for Affective Disorder.") The pineal gland and the adrenal glands share connections with a division of the nervous system called the sympathetic nervous system, in which epinephrine and norepinephrine are important neurotransmitters.

As you probably remember, levels of these neurotransmitters are thought to be abnormal in affective disorder, especially depression. These relationships give us a tantalizing glimpse into the mechanism of SAD: (1) Changes in photoperiod $\rightarrow$ (2) eyes $\rightarrow$ pineal body $\rightarrow$ (3) changes in epinephrine and norepinephrine $\rightarrow$ (4) changes in mood. This sequence is vastly oversimplified, and there

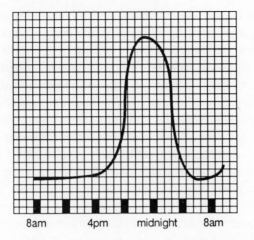

Figure 5 Production of melatonin by the pineal body over a twenty-four hour period.

are of course many, many gaps to be filled in with more research. But as with the study of poststroke depression, the study of seasonal affective disorder is providing many clues to the biological basis of mood. It is one line of research that finds links between the brain, the adrenal glands, their neurotransmitters and hormones (such as cortisol), and rhythms in mood. When the entire sequence of links is fully elucidated, we will have taken a tremendous leap forward in knowledge of the mood disorders.

The treatment of SAD with light is still being refined. The original patients were exposed to special fluorescent bulbs that reproduce closely the wavelength characteristics of sunlight. Whether ordinary artificial light is sufficient to produce the same results is not known. We know that the light must be five to ten times brighter than ordinary room light, about the same brightness as one sees looking out a window on a sunny spring day. Patients sit a few feet from a bank of lights and can read, sew, or do paperwork. They must keep their eyes open and are instructed to glance directly into the light for a few seconds every minute or so.

The timing and duration of the light exposure are also still being refined. Four to six hours of bright light each day seems necessary. Some experts feel that although it is crucial to extend the photoperiod—that is, add light hours—it doesn't matter whether the added light exposure is in the morning, in the evening, or split between the two periods. Others feel that morning light exposure is crucial for optimal response. The use of bright light treatment for depression is in its infancy; although it is more time consuming than some other treatments, it certainly has the fewest side effects.

A SAD patient treated with light notices an improvement within three or four days. Remember that antidepressant medications take two weeks at the very least to show results and even ECT often takes a week or more. The significance of this finding is unknown; it may mean that SAD symptoms are brought about by a different mechanism that responds more quickly to manipulation.

What about the patients who have summer depressions (called "reverse SAD")? One patient has been treated during the summer by exposure to cold *temperature* and had a relapse when the treatment was discontinued. Studies on temperature manipulation are in progress to see if this treatment has more potential.

Why are some people's mood disorders so closely related to photoperiod? Since we understand so little about human chronobiology—or about the mood disorders, for that matter—we don't know. The proportion of those with mood disorders who have seasonal variations is also unknown. It seems to be a minority, but the concept of SAD is so new that no good studies have yet been completed. It is intriguing to speculate that since so many people talk about "hating winter," complain of "cabin fever," and experience "spring fever," SAD may be widespread indeed. How does SAD fit into the group of mood disorders? As I said above, most SAD patients fit the profile of bipolar II (major depression and periods of mild but abnormal elation or hypomania). It may be that SAD represents a third class of mood disorders, differentiated from major depression and bipolar disorder by its timing with the seasons and its quick response to light treatment. It's plain that further study of SAD will greatly clarify the biology of mood disorders.

Schizoaffective Disorder

The DSM-III-R calls schizoaffective disorder "one of the most confusing and controversial concepts" in the classification of psychiatric illnesses. As you might guess from the word schizoaffective itself, the term is used to describe a disorder that has symptoms of both schizophrenia and affective disorder.

The symptoms of schizophrenia include prominent auditory hallucinations ("hearing voices") and bizarre thought-control experiences where patients are convinced that some outside force is controlling their thoughts, putting thoughts into their heads, or removing their thoughts. There are other bizarre symptoms as well, and none of these is often seen in mood disorders. In contrast with the symptoms of mood disorders, in schizophrenia there is usually little change in the mood state. In fact the mood appears to flatten out, and the patient seems emotionally empty—not capable of feeling either elated or depressed.

The diagnosis of schizoaffective disorder has been applied to patients who have both marked changes in mood and bizarre hallucinations and thought disruptions. The category has no treatment implications; that is, there is no specific treatment for schizoaffective disorder, and most patients who are diagnosed with this illness are treated with antipsychotic medication (the drugs used for schizophrenia), medications used for affective disorder, or a combination of both.

Some psychiatric research indicates that schizoaffective disorder is a totally separate illness, neither affective disorder nor schizophrenia. It has even been called "the third psychosis." But it seems that for every study claiming to show that schizoaffective disorder is separate, there is one claiming that patients with this disorder can always be categorized as having either schizophrenia or affective disorder and that schizoaffective disorder does not really exist as a distinct disease entity. Many experts believe schizoaffective disorder is a misleading term that has been applied to patients with severe bipolar disorder who develop bizarre symptoms when they get sick but who respond to treatments for affective disorder and so should be diagnosed as such.

It is of course theoretically possible that some people have two diseases and will therefore have symptoms of both schizophrenia and a mood disorder. Perhaps when diagnostic tests become available for mood disorders and even schizophrenia, some light will be shed on this dispute. Until then, schizoaffective disorder remains a controversial and therefore little used diagnostic category with questionable usefulness for the practicing psychiatrist.

Panic Attacks and Mood Disorders

Lisa is an interior designer who has worked for a large architectural firm for five years. She is thirty-eight but looks thirty—well-dressed, thin, vivacious, and confident.

"Dr. Knox said the quickest way for me to get rid of these attacks was to come right to you, so here I am. What do you want to know?"

It's always refreshing to see a patient I don't have to "sell" on psychiatry—someone who takes advice easily, is open and honest, and lays her cards on the table.

"I don't want to have these things happen to me again, *not one more time*. I'll do anything."

Lisa had been at a furniture show in High Point, North Carolina, when she had her first panic attack.

"I literally thought I was dying. I was walking down the aisle at the show and these terrific Italian lamps had caught my eye when I suddenly noticed that my heart was beginning to pound. 'Too much coffee, my dear,' I thought, and I started to look for the ladies' room to throw a little cold water on my face. Well the show was in this huge new exposition center for the first time this year, and I didn't know where the ladies' room was. I was heading for the information booth when it really hit me.

"My heart started pounding so hard my chest ached, and I was sure I was having a heart attack. I was dripping with sweat; my head was spinning, I couldn't breathe, my vision was going blank. I saw a chair and sat down. Well, it turned out to be a five-thousand-dollar Chippendale, so in a minute I was surrounded by security guards, and all these people were pulling at me to get out of the chair. What a nightmare! Someone, God bless him, said, 'I think she's sick.' So they laid me out on the floor, called an ambulance, and whisked me off to the hospital.

"Well, this cute paramedic was with me in the ambulance, young and strong, and he had a really calm and reassuring way about him. I was feeling better by the time I got to the hospital, and I remember thinking, 'Well, dear, this wasn't the big one after all; you've only had a *teensy* heart attack.

"When they told me they couldn't find anything, I didn't know whether to laugh or cry. I was in Dr. Knox's office the next morning, and he introduced me to the term *panic attack*. So am I going crazy or what?"

"Do you think you are?" I asked. "Sometimes people with panic attacks feel like they're losing touch with reality."

"I thought it was one of those 'near-death experiences'—you know, where people feel like they're outside their bodies, looking down on the scene as if it wasn't real."

Lisa was describing the experience of "derealization" or "depersonalization," a feeling that what's happening isn't real or that one is disconnected from the world for a moment.

She had all the symptoms of panic disorder, and the first attack at the furniture show represented what is known as the "herald" attack, which like a trumpeter announces the onset of the disorder. This first attack usually strikes without warning and takes patients completely by surprise while they are involved in some ordinary activity. The herald attack may even awaken them from sleep.

Lisa's internist had already prescribed an affective anti-anxiety medication (also called an anxiolytic medication), and she had had no recurrence of the panic symptoms in several days. Like many people who have had a panic attack, however, Lisa couldn't forget how frightening the first attack had been, and she kept worrying about having another. She started to feel anxious whenever she had to attend a trade show or some other large gathering of people, especially in an unfamiliar place. She was having what psychiatrists call "anticipatory anxiety," triggered by the thought of having another panic attack.

"I told Dr. Knox I was fine on my new medication, but he said I should come to see you at least once to find out if this Xanax is the right stuff for me. I'm not going to get hooked on this, am I?"

It was becoming clear that Lisa's "business as usual" attitude was a bit of a facade and that she had been and still was very frightened by her experience. She wasn't quite "sold" on psychiatry after all, and part of her coming to see a psychiatrist was to get a second opinion about her symptoms, which she had a hard time believing were not signs of a very serious medical or psychiatric problem. Her flippant "Am I going crazy?" expressed her real fear, and she needed more reassurance from an expert in "craziness." Her internist was astute enough to pick this up, but he realized it would be easier to get her to see a psychiatrist if he made the referral as though *he* wanted reassurance about his choice of medication.

I explained to Lisa that panic disorder is more of a biological than a psychological problem and that some people seem to have an inborn tendency toward the disorder. The herald attack certainly can be triggered by a period of stress, too much caffeine, lack of sleep, or a combination of many factors, but once it occurs it seems to turn on the tendency for more attacks. She was on exactly the medication I would have prescribed for her, and I told her she could be confident that Dr. Knox could treat her effectively. "You will get better from this," I told her.

We had a discussion of what was happening in her life now that might have triggered the attack. It turned out that her mother had died the previous month after a bout with stomach cancer. Lisa's eyes filled for a moment, but she blinked back the tears. "Don't get me started on my mother; it's a long and not very pleasant story."

Lisa had not gotten along with her mother for a long time. Her mother had had a drinking problem, and some of Lisa's childhood memories included telling lies to friends who wondered why their house was so dirty. She never endured physical or even verbal abuse, but she had been embarrassed again and again by her mother's isolation and withdrawal as she drank away the lonely afternoons in the suburbs.

"Neil says that's why I became a furniture and lamp person; I'm still obsessed with the 'house beautiful' I never lived in."

Lisa and her mother had grown further and further apart after Lisa married, and when her husband Neil was offered a job far away from Lisa's native Oregon, he took it. They had moved to the South five years ago. Lisa's mother had been diagnosed with stomach cancer only the previous summer. Lisa had made one trip back to see her mother before she died; their meeting had been strained but polite. Lisa was home with Neil when her sister called from Oregon with the news of her mother's death. Lisa didn't attend the funeral.

"You probably think that's disgraceful, but I didn't want to be a hypocrite. I had written my mother out of my life years ago, and Madeline and the rest of the family had too. I've been feeling bad about the way things turned out, but I wasn't the one who let my kids make dinner for my husband when they were six and five."

Lisa couldn't control the tears this time and took a tissue from the table in front of her.

We talked a bit more about the death, and I suggested she might get some benefit out of coming a few more times to talk and resolve her feelings better.

"I'm doing better with all that, really. I was getting over it very well until these panic attack things started, and since I've been taking my little purple pills I haven't had any more attacks. I feel much better since I've talked to you; I understand these things a lot better now. I'll stick with Dr. Knox. Thanks for seeing me."

About two weeks later I got a phone call from Lisa. She had had another panic attack—not as bad as the first, but she considered it quite a setback and was worried that her symptoms were getting worse. I saw her again in the office, and she seemed as energetic and lively as ever.

"These have got to stop. I had my period last week, and my nerves were a mess. I'm better now, but last week I completely lost my appetite and couldn't sleep. I can't keep taking pills the rest of my life every time I have my menstrual period, either!"

Like many people with anxiety, Lisa was reluctant to take her antianxiety medication regularly, so we talked about another medication approach to the treatment of panic disorder.

"Antidepressants? But I'm not depressed, I'm a nervous wreck!"

"We don't quite understand why antidepressants help with panic disorder, but they do."

It was discovered in the 1960s that some patients with severe anxiety symptoms got better when they were treated with antidepressants, especially imipramine and the MAO inhibitors. As the symptom response was investigated more thoroughly, the concept of panic disorder as a special kind of anxiety problem emerged. In patients who had discrete attacks of paralyzing anxiety separated by periods of much less anxiety or even none, the attacks seemed to be prevented by these antidepressants. Even if they were starting to have anticipatory anxiety, preventing full-blown panic attacks let them go longer without an attack, and the anticipatory anxiety gradually faded.

I explained that an antidepressant would prevent further attacks but that we would have to start her off with a small dose and gradually raise it until her symptoms responded. Unfortunately, Lisa did not tolerate imipramine well. For several weeks she tried to take it, but every time she got above twenty-five milligrams she became dizzy when she stood up and felt groggy much of the time. Even this small dose seemed to prevent the worst of the attacks, though, so I encouraged her to stay at the low dose and continue the antianxiety medication.

I told Lisa I wanted to see her in a week to assess her progress, but as before, Lisa was reluctant to see me regularly and preferred to keep in touch by phone and make an appointment only if she "needed to come in." About a month later, Lisa was back in my office.

"I'm sorry to be bothering you again, but I'm just not getting any better. I've been really thinking about myself, and I've come to the conclusion that I'm just as bad off as when I first came to see you."

Lisa had the manner of a prodigal child coming to beg forgiveness and start again on the right foot. She told me she felt tense all the time and was irritable and cross at home. Her appetite was up and down, and she had lost several pounds in the past month.

"I told you I was getting better as far as my mother was concerned. That's not true. I wake up every morning completely ashamed of myself for not having been there when she died. That part might even be getting worse; I've burst into tears at dinner twice this week for no reason."

To look at her casually, one would not suspect that Lisa was having so many symptoms, but as I looked more closely I saw her stiff posture; she was almost overcomposed, and her effort to appear calm became apparent.

It became clear to me that Lisa's panic symptoms were not the root problem. She was having a major depressive episode. She did not present the typical picture—her mood was more tense and miserable than sad—but she had vegetative symptoms and a change in self-attitude, and even her premenstrual exacerbation of symptoms was consistent with a mood disorder. Perhaps most significant, when I told her I wanted to start another antidepressant and not give up so easily this time, she agreed. "I think you're right; depression really might have been the problem all along."

We started a different antidepressant and got up to a more usual therapeutic dose in a week. In two weeks, there was no question that the diagnosis of affective disorder was the correct one.

"Now I realize why I didn't take enough of the little purple pills; I knew they weren't doing the job."

"Can you explain that to me a bit more?"

"Well, they did stop the attacks, and they made me calmer, but I realize now that I was having these bad feelings all the time that they just weren't helping with. Sometimes I began to wonder if they weren't making things worse. When my sleep started getting bad, I thought maybe I was getting dependent on them. I remember thinking, 'This is great; I'm not only a neurotic mess, I'm turning into a drug addict too.' Whatever this new stuff does, though, it's the right way to go. I haven't felt this good in months."

"Are you taking any Xanax now?"

"I haven't needed any for three days now. I'm sleeping well, and I've put on two pounds. I'm a new woman."

The relation between major depression and panic disorder is not entirely clear, but that there *is* a relationship cannot be denied. Study after study has found that patients with severe anxiety symptoms, especially panic symptoms, often also have a history of major depression. Sometimes the panic attacks occur only during the episode of depression, sometimes the two problems seem to arise independently and follow separate courses. Genetic links have also been made; that is, people with panic attacks have been found to have a higher than expected number of relatives who suffer from major depression.

The type of medications useful for treating panic disorder also points to some kind of link. Why should an antidepressant prevent anxiety symptoms? Another interesting point is the alprazolam (Lisa's purple pills), although it is in the class of other antianxiety medications (the benzodiazepine class), also has antidepressant properties. Alprazolam is structurally a little different from the other benzodiazepines (diazepam or Valium is the original benzodiazepine), and besides having some antidepressant properties, it is more effective in panic attacks than the other antianxiety drugs in its class.

Whether panic disorder and major depression are two variants of the same disorder—two sides of the same coin—is unknown. As we learn more and more about the biochemistry of both these disorders, perhaps their relationship will become clearer. In the meantime, it is important to remember that panic attacks can, in some people at least, be the first sign of the onset of a major depressive episode. Affective disorder, as we have seen, can take many forms and appear to be many different things.

Let me make a few more comments about Lisa and the problems she had in getting the right treatment. Because so many types of information are needed to make a psychiatric diagnosis, it can rarely be done in just one visit. There are always pitfalls for those who make snap judgments about diagnostic issues and are too quick to toss out information as irrelevant. Just as the psychiatrist must have an open mind whenever a new patient walks in the door, the patient needs to have an open mind as well.

Suppose when Lisa went to Dr. Knox he had taken her blood pressure and gotten 160/95. He might have said, "Lisa, this is a little worrisome. I want to see you next week so I can check this again. This may be the beginning of high blood pressure, so I want to follow up on it and not just ignore it."

Lisa most likely would have said, "Absolutely, Dr. Knox. I'll see you next week." Not, "Don't be silly; I'm too healthy to have high blood pressure. It must have been something I ate. I'll call for an appointment if I start to feel bad."

And yet that was just exactly Lisa's attitude toward her psychiatric problem. After her first visit she did not want to come back to discuss her feelings about her mother's death and explore why she had been so strongly yet unexpectedly affected by it. Later, when her symptoms were barely controlled on imipramine and alprazolam, she did not want to make regular appointments but preferred to call if she got worse (as she did).

Because affective disorder (and many other psychiatric problems as well) is very slow to develop and slow to respond to treatment, and because little guidance is available from the laboratory or X-ray department, it's vital that the patient faithfully come in for the only objective examination available to record progress or regression: the meeting with the doctor to review symptoms and progress. If Lisa had come in weekly or even biweekly, it probably would have become clear to me much sooner that she needed to be aggressively treated for affective disorder. She would have felt better sooner and in the long run would have saved herself the money she probably thought she was saving by having fewer appointments. I was reluctant to be too aggressive in switching medications because I was afraid Lisa wouldn't agree to the frequent follow-up visits she would need for me to assess progress, look for side effects, and make the necessary medication switches and dosage changes. Lisa was reluctant, and I was reluctant. What way is this to attack a health problem and get the symptoms under control as quickly as possible? Mood disorders are as serious as any other medical condition and need to be taken just as seriously. Their often slower pace is no excuse not to be vigorous in their treatment.

Lisa's case is typical in another way too. She could not take the first antidepressant but responded well to the second. This is another reason for the patient to be in close contact with the doctor and report side effects as soon as possible. There's no use waiting until the next appointment to announce, "I haven't taken the medication for a week; it made my mouth too dry." Believe me, the doctor is as interested as the patients are in their progress and wants them to get better as soon as possible. I'll discuss these issues in more detail in chapter 7.

SIX

CAUSAL FACTORS AND ASSOCIATIONS

The Heredity of Mood Disorders

A question that always comes up eventually in a discussion of mood disorders is the issue of heredity. It has been recognized for many years that mood disorders run in families, and patients are usually anxious about the chances of passing the disorder on to their offspring.

A brief discussion of the principles of genetics—the scientific study of the inheritance of biological attributes—will be useful here. The patterns and rules of inheritance in living things were first formulated by Gregor Mendel, an Austrian monk and botanist. In elegantly planned and executed experiments with plants, mostly peas, which he carried out in his monastery garden over many years, Mendel elucidated the basic principles of inheritance. Before Mendel's work in the late nineteenth century, many thought that the traits of one parent were somehow simply "blended" with the traits of the other so that any one characteristic in offspring would be intermediate between those of the two parents. Mendel, however, discovered that this was not always or even usually true. He found, for example, that crossing a pea plant that produced green peas with a plant that produced yellow ones did not produce plants with yellow-green peas (that is, an intermediate form). He found instead that *all* the seeds formed by the cross grew green peas. If he went on to cross these offspring seeds, he found that three-quarters of the second-generation seeds produced green peas and one-quarter produced yellow peas; again, there were no intermediate forms. He concluded that each parent contributed something that determined pea color, and that these "somethings" were distributed to each offspring (in this case, seeds). Most important was his discovery that although there was some interaction between them, there was no blending of traits; the seeds or offspring got either a "green" inheritance or a "yellow"; there were no "in-betweens." These "some-things" are now called "genes" and can be thought of as the units of inheritance.

Some traits seem to be determined almost completely by one gene, like the color trait in garden peas. As in the peas, knowing the pattern of these traits in the parents can permit very precise predictions about the likelihood of the offspring's inheriting a particular trait. It can often be reliably predicted that 50 percent or 25 percent (or some other simple proportion) of offspring will inherit the trait. These simple inheritance patterns are called Mendelian patterns in tribute to their discoverer.

Many human traits follow Mendelian patterns; blood types are a familiar example. Knowing both parent's blood types lets us make rather definite predictions about the blood types of their children. This is the reason blood testing can sometimes validate or invalidate paternity claims. Some human diseases seem to be passed on by a single gene that follows Mendelian patterns. Huntington's disease (or Huntington's chorea), the degenerative brain disease that killed folksinger Woody Guthrie, is an example. The children of those with Huntington's disease have a 50 percent change of developing the disease, and those that do develop it have a 50 percent chance of passing it on to a particular child. The percentages are crisp, precise, and reliable.

Most human traits, however, seem to be determined by many genes. Height is a good example. There are so many genes involved, and also so many other factors (diet, sickness, injury, and so forth) that can affect height, that predictions become very difficult to make. Tall parents have a greater chance of producing tall children than short parents do, but how many children will be taller than average and how tall they'll be is almost impossible to say.

With the development of gene-mapping techniques and extensive studies of families affected by mood disorders, we have learned much about the inheritance patterns of these illnesses. Generally speaking, mood disorders seem to fall into the category of inherited traits for which only rough estimates can be made about the chances of inheriting the illness.

People who have a first-degree relative (parent, sibling, or child) with major depression are one and one-half to three times as likely as the general population to have the disorder, and up to 25 percent of those with major depression will have a relative with a mood disorder of some kind. The hereditary occurrence of bipolar disorder is even more striking. Up to 50 percent of those with bipolar disorder have a relative with some mood disorder—ten to twenty times higher than for the general population.

Studies of twins have shed much light on the genetics of mood disorders. In identical (monozygotic) twins, which develop from the same fertilized egg and have exactly the same genes, there is a nearly 80 percent concordance rate for bipolar disorder; if one twin has bipolar disorder, there is an 80 percent chance that the other twin will have it too. Twin studies looking at major depression find high concordance rates too, but not as high as in bipolar disorder. If only one gene were involved, and if there were no environmental contribution, one would expect a 100 percent concordance rate for these disorders in identical twins. These studies seem to indicate that there is a strong genetic influence in the development of mood disorders, especially bipolar disorder, but that there are other also as yet undiscovered influences that are important in determining whether a particular individual will develop a mood disorder.

In addition to twin studies, another fertile field of endeavor in genetic research on mood disorders has been the study of Amish families. The Amish tend not to marry outside their community, so genes from outside the group that would "dilute" any genetic effect occur less frequently than in other populations. In addition, the Amish have lived for many generations in a relatively small geographical area and even today tend not to move out of that area. Therefore family Bibles, local medical records and so forth provide a lot of rather easily available information on the "pedigrees" of families. Also, as is common in many primarily agricultural societies, the Amish have many children, which makes probabilities easier to observe. (For example, an inheritance pattern where 25 percent of offspring are affected would be easier to pick up in a family with six children than in a family with two.) All of these factors make the Amish a very interesting and informative group for geneticists to study.

Psychiatric geneticists have discovered that in several Amish families bipolar disorder follows strict Mendelian inheritance patterns and seems to be caused by a single gene that can be clearly traced from generation to generation. Geneticists have also used complex statistical methods and discovered, in at least one family, exactly which of the forty-six human chromosomes carries this gene.

Other studies in non-Amish families have yielded similar results but indicate other locations for the gene. This may mean that damage to any one of several genes on different chromosomes can bring a change in the nervous system necessary and sufficient to cause bipolar disorder.

The bottom line here is that in a few extensively studied families with bipolar disorder, the inheritance pattern of the illness has been worked out well enough to permit some good predictions to be made in those families. For anyone else with a mood disorder, the predictions are much less precise. People with mood disorders, especially bipolar disorder, need to watch for the symptoms of mood problems in their families and be sure that medical treatment is not a last resort but rather first-line therapy for those who show any symptoms suggestive of mood disorders.

Another issue in the genetics of affective disorder is whether such patients have a higher than usual chance of having other psychiatric problems. Many studies have indicated that various conditions may be genetically linked in some way to affective disorder. Some researchers think alcoholism and bipolar disorder are linked, and at one time the concept was proposed that some cases of alcoholism represented "depressive spectrum disease." This idea developed from the observation that alcoholism is more common in men and major depression is more common in women. It was proposed that these two problems might represent a single disorder that was expressed differently in the two sexes, and that a single gene or set of genes was responsible that showed up in males in one form (alcoholism) and in females in another (major depression). This conclusion was supported by reports that there is an increased rate of alcoholism in male relatives of women with depression and increased rates of depression in the female relatives of alcoholic men. With extensive further study of the question, however, the theory seems to fall apart. Twin studies, and studies with more rigorous definitions of major depression, failed to confirm it, and the concept of depressive spectrum disease has fallen into disuse (see the dicussion of alcoholism and mood disorders in the next section.)

Another psychiatric problem that has been linked with affective disorder is the mysterious eating disorder anorexia nervosa. In this syndrome the patient, usually a young female, develops an abnormal fear that she is overweight and begins to lose weight through self-starvation. The symptoms of the illness sometimes include self-induced vomiting and inappropriate use of laxatives and diuretics (medications to increase urination and fluid loss). The disorder can be very difficult to treat because even at alarmingly low body weights (sometimes 70 pounds or even less), the patient continues to believe she is fat and refuses to eat. Patients with anorexia nervosa seem to have a higher than expected number of relatives with affective disorder, especially major depression. The implication is that anorexia nervosa may be a variant of affective disorder and so might be helped by the treatments available for depression.

Drug and Alcohol Abuse and Mood Disorders

To even begin to discuss drug and alcohol problems in any detail would require writing another book. Nevertheless, since the abuse of these substances is a very common problem, and since mood disorders are also relatively common, some interactions between the two are bound to occur and bear some discussion.

I said earlier that some researchers consider alcoholism another variant of affective disorder and have gone so far as to call it depressive spectrum disease. This is a highly controversial point of view, and at this time I think it's safe to say that enough genetic research contradicts the theory to conclude, at least for our discussion, that alcoholism and affective disorder are two separate problems.

A distinction still tends to be made between alcohol abuse and addiction and the abuse of and addiction to other drugs such as narcotics, cocaine, and the barbiturate sedatives. Many argue that the distinction is arbitrary and that the "choice" of whether one abuses alcohol or another drug has more to do with social and economic factors than with anything else. I'm going to lump the two problems together and call them both "chemical dependency." All theoretical considerations aside, at least two relationships between affective disorder and chemical dependency are very clear: chemical dependency can cause symptoms of affective disorder, and affective disorder can look like simple chemical dependency. Therefore discerning which disorder is at the root of a patient's symptoms can be very difficult. Nevertheless, sorting out which is the primary (first or underlying) problem and which is the secondary one is essential if the proper treatment is to be given.

Another case history will illustrate how important it is:

I was asked to consult in the care of a patient who had been admitted to the "detox" unit of a general hospital, his second detoxification admission in a month. George was a forty-five-year-old accountant for small manufacturing company who was admitted following several months of heavy alcohol use. His boss had told him that if he didn't check in to the hospital to dry out he would lose his job—period.

George was an alcoholic by just about anyone's standards. Like many men who develop alcohol problems, George had started drinking when he was a teenager. He had grown up in a small town in the South and dropped out of high school to work at a gas station just after turning seventeen. At first his drinking was not that abnormal, though it seemed to be a frequent pastime. Of course Saturday night was the time to be with his beer buddies and tie one on. And Friday, naturally, called for a few drinks to mark the end of the work week. But soon he found that the drinking that began on Friday would continue through to Saturday night without much of a break. Soon George discovered that Mondays were a lot easier to face if he just got the week started with a few beers. His drinking was a sort of joke at the gas station and even around town, where he became something of the town drunk. George started to have a harder time laughing along, however, as the years went by and he was still pumping gas at age twenty-five.

That year his alcohol use seemed to accelerate dramatically; he got into fights and spent a few nights in jail every couple of months. Then George lost his job.

This last event seemed to shock him into taking stock of his situation as he hadn't done for years. He remembered the great plans he had made as an adolescent—plans to learn auto mechanics, run his own service station, even own a chain of stations someday. But the years between those days and today seemed to have slipped away. He felt like Rip van Winkle, awakening at age twenty-five to find himself no more ready to face the future than he had been at seventeen. No job, no skills, no money, and only one friend—the bottle.

George entered an alcoholism treatment center in another town and began turning his life around. He discovered Alcoholics Anonymous. He went back to pumping gas but also got his high-school equivalency certificate, took some business courses at the community college, and found a job as a bookkeeper. He trained at night school to become an accountant and landed a "real job." He married and had children. He attended AA meetings every week for years and years and maintained total sobriety—not a single drink in nearly twenty years. He had lost the desire to drink, and he gradually dropped out of AA.

When I met George, however, he was a very sad-looking man. He sat in his darkened hospital room smoking a cigarette. His face was like a mask—grim in expression, weary. "I don't know what to tell you; I don't know how to talk to a psychiatrist. Maybe you should just ask me some questions," he said in a monotone. It was as if talking to a psychiatrist marked a new low point in his life. "Wasn't it bad enough to be a drunk? Now they think I'm crazy," he seemed to imply.

"Tell me about your slip," I said. Alcoholics Anonymous refers to an alcoholic's relapse into drinking as a "slip." The word implies something temporary, almost beyond the person's control. It was a word George would be familiar with and would show that I wasn't judging or criticizing him.

"I started feeling it come on a year ago. I should have started back with my AA meetings, but I didn't. Maybe none of this would have happened. I started having trouble at work. I couldn't concentrate; I was paranoid."

"What do you mean by that?" I asked.

"I got worried that I was making mistakes on the ledgers without realizing it. I would check and double check everything to be sure it was right. I felt sure that the company wanted to get rid of me and that the comptroller was watching my performance, gathering evidence of my incompetence so he could fire me."

"How much were you drinking at that time?"

"That was before I started drinking."

This didn't quite make sense to me. "Why did you think the company wanted to get rid of you?" I asked.

"I was sure they knew about me." Geroge looked straight at me. He seemed to be steeling himself for the inevitable next question.

"What were you sure they knew about you?"

"That I'm an alcoholic."

This was not the kind of answer I was expecting.

"I thought you said you were still sober then."

"An alcoholic is an alcoholic forever," George said, as if he were reading a death sentence.

Months before he started drinking again, George had started worrying that his somewhat disreputable past was beginning to come to light on the job where he had been a valued and productive employee for over ten years. He had been sober for so long, and had not been attending AA for so long, that he simply didn't mention it as a problem when he was hired. He had had a stable work history as an accountant for years; the remote past simply didn't figure in his hiring, and his past life as "town drunk" (even this was an overstatement) was long ago and far away. As I questioned him more closely, the symptoms of major depression came tumbling out one after another. Early morning awakening, weight loss, feelings of shame and guilt. George became convinced that his employer would "find out sooner or later anyway," so he began drinking. It was not long before the dependency syndrome became full-blown, with missed work, drinking to get started in the morning, hidden bottles at home. His wife got him to check into a detox unit of the hospital, and he seemed to make something of a turn-around. He had gone back to work but still felt tremendously insecure and had difficulty getting his work done with his usual effectiveness. He lasted only a month before he went to a bar one evening and got drunk, then called a cab and had himself driven back to the hospital. He was again admitted, but he had uncontrollable crying spells for the first two days of his hospital stay, and so his doctor ordered psychiatric consultation. I made the diagnosis of major depression complicated by alcoholism.

Did major depression cause George's alcoholism? Unfortunately, I don't think we know enough about either mood disorders or alcoholism to answer this question. I've already mentioned the controversial theory linking the two genetically. Nevertheless, some relationships between these problems are clear. I stated earlier that the drugs that are prone to abuse are those that induce some sort of euphoria or "high" in just about everyone who takes them. It is clear that some people with mood disorders will begin drinking more than usual or using other substances that induce euphoria because these chemicals temporarily relieve some of the uncomfortable feelings mood disorders cause. In depression, the slight boost in mood and feeling of relaxation caused by the rise of the alcohol level in the bloodstream may help for a while with the tension, anxiety, and pervasive gloom of the illness. Persons in the manic state may also use drugs, especially sedatives (including alcohol), to slow down their manic energy or improve their sleep. The term often used to describe this is *self-medication*. Many of these people do not suffer from chemical dependency, and when their mood disorder is properly treated they return to abstinence from drugs and more normal use of alcohol.

Nevertheless, it is clear that some people are prone to chemical dependency (which I'll continue to characterize as loss of normal behavioral restraint in the "search for the high"), and that if these people try to "treat" their mood problems with drugs or alcohol, another chain of events is set in motion that quickly causes their lives to fall apart.

I think George is one of these people. He is an alcoholic, or rather was a recovering or sober alcoholic for many years until he started to develop symptoms of major depression. Affective disorder was the banana peel he "slipped" on. If he had not gotten depressed he might not have started drinking again. He would almost certainly have stayed sober after the first detox admission given the success of treatment many years before. George's case shows how intolerable the symptoms of the depression of affective disorder can be. They can overcome even the best intentions and the strongest of wills.

When I made my diagnosis of George's problem, I broke one of my own rules, a rule I have tried to drive home to medical students and psychiatric residents for years: Diagnosis of a psychiatric problem cannot be reliably made in a substance abuser whose chemical dependency is still active. Studies indicate that between one-quarter and two-thirds of drinking alcoholics have symptoms of depression severe enough to significantly impair their everyday functioning beyond the damage caused by their intoxication and "hangovers." It is certain that not all of these people have affective disorder, even though many of them have enough symptoms of major depression that an antidepressant would certainly be prescribed by most physicians. The most effective treatment for these "secondary" depressions, however, is abstinence from alcohol. There is usually a complete resolution of the depression within several days or at most weeks after they stop drinking. Several factors made me bend my rule in George's case: he had become depressed before he started drinking, and he had remained depressed even after the first detox admission. Nevertheless, one of the leading experts on alcoholism has recently stated that in about 90 percent of patients who have symptoms of both alcoholism and depression, the depression is secondary to the alcoholism, not the other way around.*

Abuse of other drugs can also mimic the symptoms of affective disorder. Chronic marijuana abuse can cause a tired, lethargic state with low motivation that can look a lot like affective disorder. Most of the sedatives, sleeping pills, antianxiety medications, and other "downers" can cause depression in some people, sometimes even at therapeutic doses. Amphetamines or "speed" comprise a group of closely related drugs that can cause severe mood problems. These drugs are potent stimulants and produce a hyperalert, high-energy state characterized by a sense of well-being and physical robustness. As you might guess, they are very prone to abuse. Although they were widely used as appetite suppressants years ago, now they are

*M. Schuckit, "Genetic and clinical implications of alcoholism and affective disorder," in *American Journal of Psychiatry*, 143 (1986): 140–47.

prescribed rarely for some rather uncommon disorders. If any kind of medication could be called a "happy pill," the amphetamines could. Use of amphetamines can certainly induce a state that resembles hypomania, but the major problem is their tendency to cause severe depression when people who have been taking them for a while suddenly stop. The depression amphetamine withdrawal induces looks *exactly* like a major depressive episode and has caused suicides. It is interesting that amphetamines stimulate norepinephrine release in the brain. Depletion of norepinephrine may be related to major depression, and it may be that long-term use of amphetamines changes neurotransmitter receptor sensitivity in some way so that when the drug is withdrawn a state of relative norepinephrine deficiency is produced, similar to major depression. When the norepinephrine-raising property of the amphetamines was discovered, they were briefly tried as antidepressants, but results were disappointing and this use was abandoned. More recently their use in combination with traditional antidepressants has been suggested, but this use remains controversial.

Cocaine produces mood effects similar to those of amphetamines but less severe; it is far more addictive, however, perhaps accounting for its more widespread abuse.

Phencyclidine or PCP ("flakes," "angel dust") was developed as an anesthetic but produced severe psychiatric side effects during clinical trials and was never introduced for that purpose. It is used by abusers to produce hallucinatory experiences and euphoria. Many extremely violent reactions to this drug occur, some of which can be prolonged. One of the possible reactions is what has been called symptomatic mania, a mental state that is indistinguishable from mania and requires treatment with lithium. I once treated a young man in whom PCP had produced a state that could only be described as religious ecstasy and that disappeared on treatment with lithium. Most PCP psychoses are not nearly so pleasant, and suicide and grotesque murders have been reported in every city where PCP abuse has been at all prevalent.

What conclusions should we draw about the relation between affective disorder and drug and alcohol abuse? I'll quote the general rule again: The diagnosis of a psychiatric illness, perhaps especially affective disorder, cannot be reliably made in a chemically dependent person. Drugs, especially alcohol, can mimic too many of the symptoms of affective disorder. Once the chemical dependency has been treated and the effects of the drug are gone, in a small minority of persons an underlying mood disorder may be revealed that also requires treatment. However, self-medication has probably been overused to avoid treatment for what is really a much more difficult problem than mood disorders—chemical dependency.

Medical Causes of Mood Disorders

Just as many conditions can cause a symptom like shortness of breath or chest pain, many different conditions can cause the collection of symptoms that form the clinical picture of affective disorder. Various diseases, medications, poisonous substances, and infectious agents can cause the same set of biological changes in the brain as affective disorder. Both major depression and the manic state can be mimicked by several medical problems.

When patients have all the symptoms of affective disorder but it is discovered that an underlying disease or a medication is the cause of the problem, they are said to have an organic affective syndrome. Two of these words are familiar to you by now; *affective* refers to the mood, and a *syndrome* is a collection of symptoms and signs of illness that frequently occur together and are recognizable as a unique clinical entity with a limited number of causes. *Organic* is an older term in psychiatry that has already fallen out of favor to some extent but it still is used to describe psychiatric symptoms caused by an underlying "medical" problem. The dictionary defines organic as "of or arising from a bodily organ." You can see, I hope, why this is a problematic term now. It was useful when psychiatry made a clear distinction between psychological disorders, which were "of the mind," and organic disorders, which were "of the body." Depression was of the body if it was caused by a tumor, infection, hormone imbalance, or other pathological condition that could be seen on an X ray or measured with a blood test. Now that we know that major depression and bipolar disorders are associated with chemical changes in the brain and are therefore just as organic as any other disease, the term *organic affective syndrome* should probably be applied to these illnesses as well. Nevertheless, until a better term is agreed on, it remains the label applied to a major depression or manic state caused by a poison, medication, or some underlying alteration in biological function of an organ other than the brain. I'll separate the organic or medical causes of affective symptoms into several categories and describe each in turn.

Medications and Other Chemical Substances

Many medications can cause mood syndromes; in fact, we have already heard about two. Remember from chapter 1 that the observation that reserpine, the antihypertensive (high blood pressure) medication, causes symptoms of major depression practically started the biological revolution in psychiatry when it was also noted to deplete the neurotransmitter norepinephrine in nerve cells. The tendency to trigger symptoms of major depression is shared by many drugs used to treat high blood pressure.

Norepinephrine, one of the neurotransmitters intimately involved in mood, is chemically related to epinephrine, also known as adrenaline. Both these substances regulate blood pressure as well. Some blood pressure medications work by blocking the blood-vessel receptors for these substances (the adrenergic receptors), and it is these drugs that are especially likely to cause symptoms of major depression. More recently, a class of antihypertensive medications has been developed that are thought to block only the adrenergic receptors on blood vessels, the beta-adrenergic receptors. The medications are called beta-blockers (β-blockers). These are less likely to cause symptoms of major depression, but they do so in some people nonetheless.

In the section in chapter 3 titled "Complicated Depression" I told you about a patient who developed a serious depression while taking a steroid medication. This large group of medications can cause severe mood symptoms. The word *steroid* refers to a chemical structure shared by many hormones, including the sex hormones. The term *steroid medication*, however, usually refers to preparations and derivatives of cortisol, the steroid hormone secreted by the adrenal glands. Because they are potent anti-inflammatory agents, the steroids have many uses in medicine; in fact, when the first steroids became available they seemed to be miracle drugs because they are helpful in so many chronic inflammatory diseases that at the time had few effective treatments. Diseases of the joints such as rheumatoid arthritis, inflammatory diseases of the blood vessels such as lupus erythematosus and polyarteritis, bowel diseases such as ulcerative colitis and Crohn's disease, lung diseases such as chronic bronchitis, emphysema, and asthma—the list goes on and on. Steroids are also used in chemotherapy for some cancers of the blood cells and immune system.

Steroids can cause mood changes in either "direction"—that is, cause either depression or euphoria. In fact they usually cause both in a particular pattern. When first started on a steroid, the patient experiences a hypomanic state—high energy, euphoria, decreased need for sleep, and so forth. This lasts a few days until there is a gradual slipping away of these good feelings and depression sets in. The depression can range in severity from mild to severe.

Another class of medications related to the steroids are oral contraceptives. The female sex hormones are very closely related to cortisol and technically should be designated steroids, though they are not usually called that. They form the constituents of all oral contraceptives and can certainly cause mood problems, usually depression.

Another set of medications that frequently cause mood symptoms are the sedatives, often used to treat anxiety symptoms (anxiolytic medications) and to induce sleep (hypnotic medications). Older, now obsolete sedatives were especially likely to cause depression. These include the barbiturates (Nembutal, Seconal, and others), meprobamate (Miltown, Equanil), ethchlorvynol (Placidyl), and methaqualone (Quaaludes), some of them still occasionally prescribed. Even the safer, more effective medications that replaced them—drugs in the benzodiazepine class—can cause depression in some people. These medications include diazepam (Valium), alprazolam (Xanax), and others. All these medications seem to have at least some affinity with alcohol and may cause depression for the same reasons. They are also prone to abuse, sometimes making matters worse. (For a full discussion of these issues see the section in this chapter, "Drug and Alcohol Abuse and Mood Disorders.")

There are a few poisons that can cause mood disorders. They usually cause many other problems and quickly make themselves known with other symptoms, but if the patient is exposed to low levels over a long period, depression may be the only symptom for quite a while, leading to diagnostic confusion.

One poisonous substance that can cause depression and to which long-term low-level exposure is not rare is lead. Painters who inhale lead from paint dust or burning old paint can be exposed to toxic levels and show all the symptoms of major depression— low mood, fatigue, irritability, loss of interest in sex, and so on. In a study of 30 men exposed to lead and evaluated at an occupational medicine clinic, most complained of depression among other symptoms, and several reported that depressed mood was their most severe symptom. One patient had complete resolution of his depression when treated with a lead-removing medication but had a full relapse when he resumed scraping and sanding paint without a face mask.*

Hormonal Imbalances

In the previous section I noted that steroid medications can cause mood problems, so it should come as no surprise that medical problems that affect the amount of steroids the adrenal glands produce can also cause mood disorders. Tumors of the adrenals can sometimes cause them to secrete hormones in abnormally large amounts, producing essentially the same result as taking steroid medication. Though it may seem paradoxical, a deficiency of steroid hormones can also cause mood symptoms. This can occur when adrenal gland tissue is destroyed by tumor or infection. Sometimes the adrenal glands seem to shrivel up for no apparent reason, a condition known as Addison's disease. A lack of the hormones secreted by the adrenals can produce a generalized weakness, loss of appetite, weight loss, and other symptoms that can mimic major depression.

Mood seems to be even more closely tied to the thyroid system. The details of the link between the thyroid hormones and mood are not entirely clear, but several facts are pretty much proved. Hypothyroidism (*hypo-* meaning low) can clearly cause all the symptoms of major depression. Patients can experience slowed thinking, a decreased energy level, and memory problems in addition to depressed mood, which is sometimes of suicidal proportions.

In some people who suffer depressive symptoms that seem to

*R. S. Schottenfield, and M. R. Culen, "Organic affective illness associated with lead intoxication," in *American Journal of Psychiatry* 141 (1984): 1423-26.

be caused by thyroid malfunction, laboratory tests of thyroid function seem to be normal. These patients get better when they are treated with thyroid hormones even though their test results do not indicate thyroid problems. Sometimes a depression that responds incompletely to the usual treatment with antidepressants can become fully responsive if a small amount of thyroid hormones is added to the antidepressant. Whether these patients suffer from some subtle deficiency of thyroid hormone incapable of being measured or whether they have a variant of major depression that is more dependent on thyroid hormones for its expression remains to be seen.

I'll pause here for a moment to say that the connections between these two hormonal systems, adrenal and thyroid, seem to be very important in the development of the symptoms of affective disorder. I've already mentioned that the pattern of secretion of the adrenal hormones is disrupted in some persons with major depression (see "Tests for Affective Disorder" in chapter 3), and that too much or too little of the adrenal steroid hormones, which may be caused by adrenal gland disease, can mimic all the symptoms of hypomania and depression.

Too little of the thyroid hormones can mimic the symptoms of depression, and sometimes extra thyroid hormones must be added to antidepressants to completely relieve symptoms. Without going into unnecessary detail, let me state that the activity of both the adrenals and the thyroid glands is regulated by the pituitary gland at the base of the brain, and that the pituitary in turn receives hormonal and possibly neural input from a part of the brain called the hypothalamus. As with the pineal body, melatonin, and light and their effects on mood (see "Seasonal Affective Disorder" in chapter 5), the facts about the thyroid and adrenal glands, the effect of their hormones on mood, and their connections to the brain offer some tantalizing room for speculation about the nature and ultimate causes of the mood disorders and will no doubt shed much light on the search for causes and better treatments.

A rarer hormonal problem that can cause mood changes is disease of the parathyroid. The parathyroid glands control the level of calcium in the bloodstream, and it is the abnormal calcium level that seems to cause the mood problems. Too much calcium can cause depression; too little causes a severe anxiety state that can also look like major depression of the more "agitated" type.

Other Nervous System Diseases

Several other illnesses can include prominent mood disturbances as part of their symptom picture. First, there are several illnesses that also affect the brain and cause degeneration of particular centers. Patients with Parkinson's disease, a slowly degenerative movement disorder, can sometimes have episodes of major depression in the course of their illness, and in Huntington's disease, a devastating degenerative disorder that affects movement and causes dementia, an episode of affective disorder may be the first symptom. In Huntington's there is usually a family history of the illness, which is a tip-off to the diagnosis of the underlying disorder.

Multiple sclerosis, a puzzling nervous-system disease in which there is spotty, unpredictable destruction of neural tissue, can cause mood changes either early in the disease or late in its course.

Very rarely, brain tumors can present as mood disturbances alone; like the other illnesses, they do not remain "silent" for long, and soon other symptoms like seizures and paralysis occur and point to the underlying disorder.

Infections

A whole range of infections have been implicated as possibly causing mood disturbances, especially depression. Depression associated with tuberculosis has been known for many years, but since this illness has fortunately become rare in this country, so has the associated depression. There is an association between certain viral infections and depression as well. Patients with hepatitis, a viral infection of the liver, and with mononucleosis, an often lengthy viral infection that causes profound fatigue, often complain of depression.

More recently a syndrome has been described that is thought to be caused by the same virus that causes mononucleosis, the Epstein-Barr virus. Patients have recurrent bouts of fatigue, weight loss, low mood, sleep disturbances, trouble in concentrating, and other symptoms. The syndrome has also been called chronic viral fatigue syndrome and has sparked a great deal of debate about the connection between the functioning of the immune system and mood disorders.

Other Conditions

An association has long been reported between abdominal malignancies, especially cancer of the pancreas, and major depression. The mechanism for this is completely unknown, but complaints of depression for several months before the other symptoms of the disease emerge have been observed too often to be explained simply as a coincidence.

Vitamin deficiencies can cause depression, but true vitamin deficienceis are rare and have many associated symptoms, so the misdiagnosis of affective disorder in such cases would be unlikely.

One has only to scan psychiatric journals for a few months to read reports associating the symptoms of affective disorder with what can seem like every medication, poison, and disease known to medicine. What does it all mean? For the neuroscientist, every association may be another piece in the puzzle of affective disorder, but for practicing psychiatrists and their patients the picture can be very confusing. If so many diseases, deficiencies, and metabolic disturbances can mimic mood disorders, how much testing for underlying disease should be done? Can we distill some practical guidelines on the diagnosis and treatment of mood disorders from all the data on associated conditions?

Perhaps the first point to make is that affective disorder *is* very common, and that the one "underlying" disorder that often turns up to look like affective disorder is alcohol abuse. Sheer numerical probability makes it likely that the diagnosis of affective disorder in a person with the symptoms of that disorder is correct. (There's an old folk-saying in medicine: "If you hear the sound of hoofbeats, don't look for zebras.")

Second, it is rare for a mood change and other symptoms of a mood disorder to be the *only* signs of a serious underlying illness. People with thyroid problems have changes in pulse rate, body weight, and skin texture. Those with too much steroid circulating have alterations in the distribution of body fat and other symptoms. People with infections run fevers. The list goes on and on. Even if the mood change is at first the only symptom, the others will follow in time, and the diagnosis will become clear.

Third, a mood disorder that is caused by another underlying

illness often will not respond well to the usual treatments. Antidepressants or lithium will not "coverup" symptoms and allow an undiagnosed medical problem to worsen. If the problem is not affective disorder, treatments for affective disorder tend not to produce good results.

It is simply not sound medical practice to try to track down every possible "medical" cause of mood disturbances before starting treatment, especially since the treatment of mood disorders is so benign and effective. If all the patients who complain of depression were given a total body CAT scan, had every hormone measured, were tested for lead, aresenic, and mercury, and were otherwise evaluated for every medical condition associated with mood changes, not only would they lose a lot of blood, collect gallons of urine, and be exposed to unnecessary radiation (not to mention get a huge bill!), it would be months before they got any treatment.

(Nevertheless, medical problems do sometimes turn out to be present, and thus it is important to have medical input into the treatment process, especially in the beginning. See "Who Can Help" in chapter 7.)

Sleep and Depression

Just as the relations observed between light and mood in seasonal affective disorder and between stroke and depression have taught neuroscientists a great deal about affective disorder, study of the relation between sleep and mood disorders has been very fruitful in understanding both the normal experience of sleep and the abnormal experiences of patients with mood disorders. The study of sleep has even indicated some very promising new treatment approaches to affective disorder.

Over twenty years ago, serious study of sleep revealed that it is a very complicated process consisting of many stages and levels. It had previously been thought that sleep was simply a time of little or no activity, either physical or mental. Various explanations were offered for the process of dreaming (which certainly is a mental activity occurring during sleep), but the sleeping person seemed to be more or less like a machine that had been turned off, especially as far as mental activity was concerned.

The tool that has been used most effectively to investigate sleep is the electroencephalogram (EEG), *electro-* referring to electricity, *encephalo-* referring to the brain, and *-gram* meaning a written record. When an EEG is performed, electrodes, which can measure small amounts of electricity much as sensitive microphones pick up faint sounds, are placed around the person's scalp. Two electrodes are also placed near the temples to measure eye movements. The process and equipment are just like those used in the more familiar electrocardiogram, or EKG.

Unlike the heart, though, which has a relatively simple pattern of electrical activity, the brain produces electrical activity that is monumentally complex. The EEG can gather only the vaguest data about the activity of the brain; as a diagnostic tool, it can pick up a few types of abnormalities like large tumors or seizure activity. And although it is sensitive, it is not very specific in indicating the type of problem present. Because of this specificity problem, interpreting the EEG is tricky; I tell medical students it's like trying to diagnose car trouble by listening to the engine: even an amateur can tell when something is really wrong, but only experts can be specific about the nature of the problem, and even they must guess.

Fortunately, though, although the EEG can reveal little about the type of brain activity going on, it gives a rather good measurement of the *level* of activity, and this is why it has proved so useful in studying sleep. When EEGs were run on sleeping persons throughout the night, it became clear that far from constituting a simple switch from high brain activity to low, sleep consisted of many stages of different levels of activity, and during some of them the brain seemed just as active as in the waking state. There was consistency in the pattern as well, and the term *sleep architecture* was coined to denote the pattern of brain activity throughout the night.

It's not necessary to go into much detail about sleep architecture, but I do want to mention several stages that are important. After falling asleep, a person passes through lighter and then progressively deeper levels of sleep when the brain seems to slow down and become quiescent. Other body activities slow too. For example, the heartbeat and blood pressure drop to the lowest levels of the twenty-four-hour day. The process is like a submarine descending to darker, quieter, deeper water. The deepest stage is called slow wave sleep (SWS) after the type of EEG waves that characterize it. SWS is thought to be the physically restorative part of sleep;

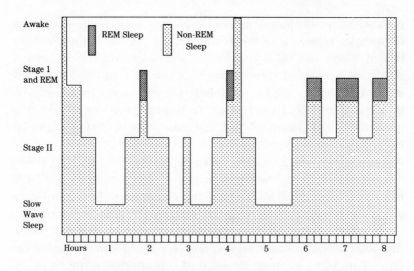

Figure 6   Typical Sleep Pattern of a Young Adult

in sleep experiments people who were awakened every time they entered SWS but were allowed to experience the other stages complained of muscle aches and pains. About an hour into the cycle, the sleep "submarine" starts to rise again, and the EEG indicates brain activity not too different from wakefulness. Nevertheless, the person is still asleep, and in fact this is when dreaming occurs. The eyes can be seen moving beneath closed lids, a characteristic that gives this stage of sleep its name: rapid eye movement or REM sleep. The function of REM sleep is not known. It has been speculated that it is somehow necessary for the development of the memory for the day's events, but this is far from certain. People who are REM deprived become irritable and even agitated.

During the night the level of sleep rises and falls; the length of each cycle and the amount of SWS and REM sleep stay within certain normal ranges in healthy persons of given ages who are then said to have normal sleep architecture (see fig. 6).

One of the hallmarks of major depression is sleep disturbance, and the EEG reveals that a depressed person's sleep architecture is indeed abnormal in several ways. In depression, less of the time asleep is spent in SWS. Since this is the deep, restorative part of sleep, this change may explain the "restless" quality of the depressed person's sleep. The duration and intensity of REM sleep are greater in depressed people, and they enter the first REM stage sooner after falling asleep, a condition known as "short REM latency."

When this change in the sleep architecture was first observed and the findings were shown to be relatively consistent, it seemed that a test for major depression might have been discovered. But just as with the dexamethasone suppression test (see "Tests for Affective Disorder" in chapter 3), similar findings were found too often in nondepressed persons for the change to be of much use as a diagnostic tool. Nevertheless the findings are consistent enough in enough depressed patients to have caused a great deal of scientific interest in the interrelations between sleep and depression.

Sleep study has led to new treatments for depression, too. About fifteen years ago there were several reports of patients with major depression who had an improvement in mood if they were deprived of sleep. Study after study has replicated this finding: if depressed persons are kept awake all night, their mood is much better the next day. Although the improvement is long lasting in a few patients, most have a relapse of their depressed mood as soon as they get some sleep. Several manipulations of sleep, such as sleep deprivation for only part of the night, have been tried and offer some further benefit, since partial sleep deprivation can be used several nights in a row. It appears that deprivation in the latter part of the night alone may be as effective as total sleep deprivation. Since more time is spent in REM sleep during this part of the night, some have speculated that REM deprivation is the key. Another concept is that of "phase advance." In this technique patients go to sleep five hours or so earlier than normal and awaken comparably earlier. Thus they are not acutally deprived of sleep, and the treatment can be carried out almost indefinitely. Again, since depressed persons have short REM latency—that is, they go into REM sleep earlier in the night than normal sleepers—the theory is that by going to sleep sooner they are forcing their abnormal sleep architecture into a more normal pattern. Combination of sleep deprivation or phase advance and medications are being investigated as well and perhaps hold the most promise.

As in seasonal affective disorder and light treatment, the details of a consistently effective technique that is not too difficult for patients to perform have not yet been worked out. Nevertheless, sleep manipulation shows great promise as an additional way to treat depression or a way to make medications for depression work faster or better.

Another discovery is that sleep deprivation can precipitate manic episodes in patients with bipolar disorder. This has very important implications in that it suggests that by observing regular bedtimes bipolar patients may reduce the risk of an episode of mania.

As in seasonal affective disorder, all this work seems to indicate some sort of connection between mood regulation and an internal clock. It may be that by learning to manipulate this clock we will be able to provide symptom relief more quickly, with less medication or perhaps no medication at all.

PART THREE

Getting Better

SEVEN

ADVICE FOR MOOD DISORDER PATIENTS AND THEIR FAMILIES

In the preceding chapters I have spent a lot of time explaining what the mood disorders are, how to recognize their symptoms, and how they are treated, as well as describing some of their many variations. Now I shall give what I hope is some practical advice to those who have mood disorders and to their families.

First I shall present a guide to getting the proper treatment. Many people seem to feel that seeing a psychiatrist is a desperate last resort when all else fails. I want to persuade you that consulting a psychiatrist for symptoms of depression is as logical as consulting a cardiologist about chest pains or an ophthalmologist about eye problems.

In the section called "Living with a Mood Disorder," I'll address practical issues such as relapse.

Since psychotherapy is such an important part of what psychiatrists do, and such a necessary part of the treatment of mood disorders, I'll spend some time exploring this very special and useful type of treatment.

Sometimes, when symptoms are severe, hospitalization is indicated. Like ECT, this very valuable aspect of the treatment of mood disorders is often feared and resisted because of misconceptions based on outdated ideas. I'll explain what hospitalization in a modern psychiatric unit is like.

Finally, I'll comment on the very real problem of the stigma associated with psychiatric illness and psychiatric treatment.

Who Can Help? The Mental Health Professionals

Does everyone who may be suffering from a mood disorder need to see a psychiatrist? Believe it or not, there is some disagreement about this. Much of the disagreement comes from nonpsychiatrist practitioners who feel they are just as qualified and competent to treat mood problems as a psychiatrist is. In some cases they are right. To address this issue, let's survey the various professionals who treat psychiatric problems.

Psychiatrists

As you have read the foregoing chapters, you will have gotten some idea what treatment from a psychiatrist is like. Many of those who come to my office for help have terrible notions about psychiatrists. Depending on their exposure to the profession and the media protrayals they have seen, they may expect a monster intent on locking them up or, perhaps more frequently, an aloof, slightly bizarre, bearded character capable of discerning their deepest, darkest secrets from the way they say hello.

Perhaps the most important fact to remember, and the thing that separates psychiatrists from all the other mental health professionals, is that a psychiatrist is a medical doctor (M.D.). More precisely, a psychiatrist specializes in the treatment of illnesses whose symptoms involve emotion, behavior, and other disorders of mental functioning. (The word *psychiatrist* comes from *psyche*, "mind," and *iatros*, "physician." Thus a psychiatrist is a physician of the mind.)

In medical school psychiatrists have learned how to perform a physical examination, deliver babies, treat high blood pressure, look at X-rays, suture lacerations—in short, they have become familiar with many, many aspects of health and disease. After an internship that consists of at least several months of caring for patients with general medical problems, psychiatrists enter a training program to learn about the diagnosis and treatment of psychiatric problems. (The training period *after* medical school is four years.)

Remember that we deal with illnesses whose symptoms mainly concern emotion and behavior. Alzheimer's disease is a good example of a "medical" illness where the treatment consists of helping to manage behavioral problems, and a psychiatrist is often involved.

Psychiatrists are like any other doctor in most ways, and the way we do our work is rooted in the same traditions and methods of practice as for doctors in other specialties. We take a medical history, asking about when the symptoms started, the quality of symptoms, associated details, and anything that seems to make the symptoms better or worse. Patients are asked about their family history, which is important because mood problems in relatives make the diagnosis of a mood disorder more likely. We perform the equivalent of a physical exam called a mental status exam; instead of listening to the heart or otherwise examining the workings of the body, we ask patients about their mood and their anxiety feelings, and often pose a few questions to test memory and concentration. We also try to get to know patients, asking something about their family, their education, work, marriage or "significant other" relationship, and so forth. Some people think that at the first meeting the psychiatrist will want them to talk for hours in deep detail about their childhood, their sexual fantasies, and so forth. Nothing could be further from the truth. At least once a month, it seems, I see a new patient who starts off the appointment by saying something like, "I've never talked to a psychiatrist before, so I don't know what you want me to say." It's almost as if they think the psychiatrist uses some special language, or reads minds, or will try to "trick" them into revealing something they are sensitive about. Like any other doctor, the psychiatrist is interested in helping—that's what patients pay us for! We need to know what the problem is so we can work with the patient to provide relief.

I don't apologize for my use of the word *patient*, by the way. I don't have *clients*. I think a special kind of relationship exists between physician and patient that is very different from that between, say, an accountant and a client. Doctors *take care* of patients, unlike other professionals who provide services for clients.

Nonphysician Mental Health Professionals

A psychologist usually has a Ph.D. degree in psychology from a university, although anyone with any degree in psychology, a bachelor's degree or master's degree, for example, can use the title psychologist in some states. Most states have laws defining who can do so legally, as well as a licensing requirement of some type. The amount of training and experience psychologists have can thus vary quite a bit. Psychology can perhaps be defined as the science of the mind, and thus psychologists do not necessarily treat illness. Some, for example, limit themselves to research, psychological testing, IQ testing, and so forth.

Although a psychologist who has a Ph.D. can use the title doctor, psychologists are not medical doctors and thus cannot prescribe medicine, perform physical examinations, or order and interpret laboratory tests. They have not treated medical problems as part of their training, and many are totally unfamiliar with the biological factors that can cause mood problems.

There are also other mental health professionals who may see people with mood disorders. Social workers have often studied counseling, especially family counseling. Formerly social workers were much involved with "social welfare" programs, but today most do much more than, say, help people get food stamps. Many schools of social work offer special tracks in counseling or clinical social work, and these programs often prepare very good psychotherapists. (See "Psychotherapy" below to see how this fits into the treatment of mood disorders.) Most social workers who see patients have master's degrees.

Nurses can specialize in psychiatric nursing and often see patients in their own practice. Most of these have also gotten master's degrees. Because nurses have a medical background, they are perhaps more familiar with the medical model and more comfortable seeing patients who are taking medication. Of course nurses cannot prescribe medication.

Clergy do pastoral counseling and usually have special training to recognize more serious problems and make the proper referrals.

Very recently, another type of mental health professional has come on the scene, the psychiatrist's assistant. Like the more familiar physician's assistant, these professionals receive in-depth training in psychiatric illnesses, psychiatric medications, and other aspects of psychiatry so that they can, under the direct supervision of the psychiatrist, perform some of the more routine aspects of psychiatric care. This may consist, for example, of seeing patients who are doing well on lithium, asking about symptoms and side effects, ordering lab tests, and presenting this information to the psychiatrist for review and treatment decisions.

Later in this chapter I will discuss the role of counseling and psychotherapy in the treatment of mood disorders. As will become clear, having an M.D. or even being a psychiatrist does not necessarily make one a skilled psychotherapist, and many nonphysicians are expert at this type of treatment. (By the way, anyone who does psychotherapy is called a psychotherapist; this title implies nothing about training or educational background.) Nevertheless, all the nonphysician professionals lack the training to treat affective disorder *by themselves*, for though many may have gained experience working in a psychiatric hospital or with a psychiatrist, the fact remains that they cannot perform the treatment that is often the crucial intervention in mood disorders—prescribing medication.

Family Practice Physicians

Several years ago, family practice came into being as a separate medical speciality. A family practitioner is a medical doctor who emphasizes knowing enough about all branches of medicine to treat most common medical problems competently. In a sense the family practitioner's specialty is not being too specialized. It may seem that a family practitioner would not be very knowledgeable about mood disorders, but this is not so. Remember that their training readies family practitioners to treat *common* medical problems, and mood disorders are certainly very common. In my experience, among all the medical specialists (other than psychiatrists, of course) family practitioners are the most experienced and competent when it comes to treating patients with psychiatric problems. Although many do not call themselves that, most doctors who practice general internal medicine are like family practitioners in many ways and also usually have a great deal of experience with mood disorders.

A word here about the psychoanalyst. It is a common misconception that every psychiatrist is a psychoanalyst—even that anyone who talks to people about their emotional symptoms, trying to figure out the problem and help with it, is "psychoanalyzing" them. A psychoanalyst, usually referred to simply as an analyst, practices an extremely specialized type of psychotherapy based on the theories of the great psychiatrist Sigmund Freud. Most analysts are M.D.'s who have completed a residency in psychiatry and have then entered a lengthy training period at a psychoanalytic institute where they study the theories of Freud and of subsequent practitioners who elaborated on and further developed Freud's theory. This body of knowledge is collectively known as psychoanalytic theory, and the type of psychotherapy that follows these principles is called psychoanalysis or simply analysis. Analysis is a long, very intensive type of treatment in which the patient lies on the famous couch and the analyst sits behind it. Patients in analysis see their therapists three or four times a week for an hour, and the complex task of a very deep, detailed exploration of the patient's entire life experience and personality takes years. Only a minority of psychiatrists are analysts, and most of these have only a few of their patients in analysis. The vast majority of patients who see psychiatrists have sessions not very different from their appointments with their medical doctors.

You can see that the question posed in the title of this section is not a simple one. There is a wide range of knowledgeable people who can help greatly in the treatment of mood disorders. So where does one begin to look for help? Let's limit ourselves here to a discussion of depression, since it is by far the most common mood symptom. Since not all depression is due to affective disorder (see "Other Types of Depression" in chapter 2), sometimes psychotherapy, counseling, or just good advice may be all that's required to treat the problem.

Perhaps rather than trying to answer Who can help? it would be more useful to discuss who can best decide on the most appropriate treatment when a person is having depression, mood swings, or other mood problems. I think the answer is clear. The first person to be consulted for evaluation of a possible mood disorder should be an M.D. Some will disagree with me about this, but if you review

"Medical Causes of Mood Disorders" in chapter 6, you'll see why I think it is necessary. No matter how well trained and experienced a psychologist, social worker, or even a nurse may be, many simply do not have the familiarity with medical problems that an M.D. does.

Most general and family practitioners will be able to treat less severe mood disorders quite well; they *want* to do so as part of their commitment to providing as much of their patients' care as possible. In fact, since people with mood disorders are so common, there simply aren't enough psychiatrists to treat them all. Besides, it's always best if one can receive treatment from the doctor who knows one's history rather than from a new and unfamiliar doctor, even a specialist. Those who have family doctors should see them first. If more specialized care is needed, family practitioners will be able to recommend psychiatrists they have confidence in, and therefore the patient will feel confident too. If the person with symptoms of a mood disorder does not have a family doctor, there's a lot to be said for seeing a psychiatrist first. After all, psychiatrists see and treat mood disorders much more frequently than other doctors and are the most knowledgeable and experienced experts available.

In the case of bipolar disorder, there is much to be said for not settling for anyone other than a psychiatrist. The medical treatment of bipolar disorder can be more complicated. Physicians in other specialties will probably have little experience with prescribing lithium and may not know how to handle its side effects as well as a psychiatrist. Also, of all the medicines for treating mood disorders, those used in bipolar disorder seem to keep changing the fastest. For example, in the past five years or so the use of the anticonvulsant medications in bipolar disorder has dramatically increased. The most up-to-date treatment of bipolar disorder seems to go out of date very quickly, and only a psychiatrist usually has time to monitor the latest information; most other specialists are too busy keeping up with their own rapidly changing specialities.

I have not tried to list national experts in the field of mood disorders, for several reasons. First of all, very few people need a "super doctor." Most simply need a good psychiatrist who is up to date on the treatment of mood disorders. Second, the "super docs" move around a lot; they may switch from clinical work to spending a year just doing research and not seeing patients, so a list of where they are and who is seeing patients quickly becomes obsolete. Instead, I want to give advice on finding a doctor in the community who is right for the patient—advice that will not go out of date as a list of names does.

As in choosing any physician, it is important to pick a psychiatrist the patient feels completely comfortable with. Recommendations from friends, relatives, and of course the family doctor are a good way to find a good match. I don't think patients should be made to apologize for preferring, say, a female rather than a male psychiatrist, although some experts believe such preferences should not be honored. The psychiatrist will be a psychotherapist too, and there has always been a debate in the psychotherapy literature on whether such preferences indicate "neurotic" patterns that need to be challenged and worked through. There has been no conclusive research to answer this question, but my own thinking is that time spent working through these issues is time wasted in treating the medical problem of mood disease. The sooner the patient feels totally comfortable with the psychiatrist, the sooner the real problem—the mood disorder—can be tackled.

If friends and family can't make a referral and there is no family doctor, call the local Mental Health Association, which usually has a list of good psychiatrists. Hospitals often have physician referral services too. If your town has a university with a medical school, there will be a department of psychiatry and often a faculty practice group. Don't be afraid to request a doctor who is male or female. Many psychiatrists also identify themselves as serving blacks, Hispanics, and other ethnic groups, as being affirmative of gay and lesbian orientation, and so forth. Often a community center has a list of doctors who serve the community, and this can be a resource. We are fortunate in this country to have community mental health centers serving almost every community. Their mandate from state, county, or other municipalities is to provide high-quality mental health care to all who apply for it, regardless of ability to pay. When finances are a problem, this is a valuable resource. The local community mental health center will also usually have a list of private-practice psychiatrists as well and will be glad to make a referral.

As with any medical problem, don't hesitate to get another opinion or to switch doctors if your needs are not being met or if the treating physician doesn't seem responsive enough.

Living with a Mood Disorder

People never like to be told they have an illness, even one that is treatable. In many ways mood disorders are crueler in their effect on their victim than any other chronic medical condition because of the way they mimic normal functioning—normal changes in mood. Living with a mood disorder is trying for both sufferers and their families. This section will address some of the problems both groups have in living with a mood disorder.

Relapse

Patients often ask me, "Will I need to take medication the rest of my life?" From the chapters on treatment, you have seen that mood disorders are episodic and that often, especially in major depression, the periods of remission can be long. Even in bipolar disorder there may be months or years between episodes. Yet the onset of an episode can be sudden, sometimes so sudden that there is not enough time to prevent some very uncomfortable symptoms that may persist for days or even weeks before treatment takes effect. Unfortunately there is no test (yet) the sufferer can have done, say, every six months to see if an episode of mood disorder is beginning. Thus the patient who is not on medication must be vigilant to detect signs of recurrence.

In both major depression and bipolar disorder, sleep disturbance is often the earliest sign. If sleep problems persist more than a few days for no apparent reason, it's a good idea to get in touch with the treating physician. I mentioned in the section on sleep that sleep deprivation is thought to precipitate manic episodes in bipolar disorder. Some experts believe that keeping the biological clock "tuned" by regular bedtimes and arising times is extremely important in the control of mood symptoms. "Regularizing" one's life is one way to reduce many types of physical and mental stress and may lessen the chance of relapse.

Energy-level changes can also be an early sign of relapse. Low energy, fatigue, and lack of interest in school or work can be early signs of depression, and increased energy or decreased desire to rest and sleep can herald the onset of hypomania or the manic state. Family members are often the most accurate monitors. Those with mood disorders should resist the temptation to explain away exaggerated changes in mood that their families notice. Just as patients are often the last ones to see improvement after medication is started for depression, they may be the last to realize that an episode of mood disorder is beginning. In patients I have come to know well, I can notice small things like tenseness in the facial muscles and changes in posture that indicate the onset of an episode before the patients realize what is happening. Family members can often pick up these changes even earlier, and they bear listening to—by both the patient and the doctor.

There is a fine line, however, between this type of vigilance and an obsessive scrutiny of the patient's every thought and feeling. It can be very destructive and demoralizing to have someone ask, "Are you taking your medication?" every time one shows disappointment or enthusiasm over something. Having a mood disorder does not mean every change in mood might be abnormal.

Once they are correctly diagnosed and treated, most people with mood disorders quickly learn to differentiate between normal and abnormal feelings and thoughts. Many of my patients, even before they knew they were having episodes of affective disorder, have had names for their episodes: "my gloomy spells," "my hyper days," and so forth. Once they understand the illness and, even more important, see the symptoms fade away with treatment, it's not difficult to recognize particular symptoms. As I said earlier, many patients can identify symptoms that are almost earmarks of their episodes. "Whenever I find myself thinking about my grandmother's death and feeling guilty about it, I *know* it's starting," one of my patients once told me. The wife of one of my patients could tell when her husband was starting to have a manic episode by the number of phone calls he made. What is important is to pay serious attention to these symptoms and get the proper medical attention. Just as the heart patient who wants to stay well will never ignore chest pain and the diabetic patient knows the symptoms of high blood sugar, the mood disorder patient should know the symptoms of relapse and get in touch with the doctor immediately when they occur.

If the mood disorder patient who is not on medication should be especially vigilant for the appearance of symptoms, why stop taking medication? This is a very personal decision that should be made with great care and after talking at length with the doctor. Naturally no one likes to take medication, but it is the single most important step one can take to minimize the chance of relapse.

Some people say they resent having to take a medication that "controls" them. This is simply the wrong way to look at it. Antidepressants and lithium can no more "control" a person with a mood disorder than insulin "controls" a diabetic. On the contrary, just as diabetics use insulin to control their illness, these medications put patients back in control of their lives rather than at the mercy of the disease.

Medication Issues

Medication is such an important part of the treatment of mood disorders that I shall make some general points about taking medicine and also reiterate some things about specific drugs used to treat mood disorders.

First, it is vital that patients be honest with the physician about taking or not taking medication. Some seem afraid to tell their doctors about side effects or to say a medication is not working as expected. They think their doctors will be disappointed in them or get angry if they complain about their medication. I would rather get a phone call one week into the treatment from a patient worried about a side effect than see that person at the next appointment and hear, "I only took the medication one day; it made me feel funny, so I stopped it two weeks ago." Now that *will* make me angry!

Another point is that feeling back to normal does *not* mean the need for medication is over. Remember, unlike some other illnesses that medication can cure, in mood disorder antidepressants and lithium *treat* the problem. They control the symptoms during the time the "mood system" isn't working correctly, and if they are stopped too soon, the symptoms can come right back. Stopping antidepressant medication or lithium less than six months after starting them places one at very high risk for relapse. Even stopping after less than a year is probably risky. Mood disorder patients should ask themselves not Why keep taking it? but rather Why *not* keep taking it? If there aren't good answers to the second question, why take the risk?

Many patients ask if they can drink alcohol while on medication. Most experts are hesitant to absolutely forbid alcohol, and I am too. But if the medication is sedating, alcohol will increase the sedative effect, and one may seem very intoxicated after a relatively small amount of alcohol. For this reason it is important to watch oneself closely and go very slowly when using alcohol for the first time while taking medication. Some drugs, like lithium, have no sedative effect, and the interaction with alcohol is not significant.

There is a broader issue concerning alcohol, however. When my patients ask, "How many drinks can I have?" I often retort, "That's like a diabetic asking how many chocolate cupcakes—the fewer the better!" Remember that alcohol is a destabilizer for the nervous system and seems to have even more of a destabilizing influence on mood.

Another issue is pregnancy and medication. It's probably a good idea for all women in the childbearing years to take precautions not to become pregnant while taking medication. This is certainly true for lithium, which has been proved to cause severe heart defects in children whose mothers became pregnant while taking it. The antidepressants have not been linked to any particular birth defects, but few reliable data are available for most of them. Remember that most of the baby's major organ systems are developing in the first few weeks after conception, usually before the mother even knows she is pregnant. This means that stopping a medication when the patient misses her period or the pregnancy test comes back positive may be too late to prevent severe birth defects. Preventing conception while taking medication is the key. Often pregnant women can go back on their mood disorder medication later in the pregnancy and come off it shortly before their due date (to avoid any sedation of the newborn). The patient who wants to conceive always needs to have a discussion with her doctor before stopping medication. Stopping medication has risks too—the risk of relapse. Just as the "medically" ill woman's pregnancy is risky, the depressed, and especially the manic, woman is at a higher risk than her peers for problems in pregnancy.

The exact timing of taking these drugs is usually not crucial. All the antidepressants build up in the body slowly and are removed slowly. For this reason it is not necessary to take the medicine several times a day; the entire dose can usually be taken at one time. This also means that taking these medications at a particular time of day is not usually important, although many of the sedating antidepressants are taken at night to promote sleep. It is probably not necessary to "double up" if one misses a dose of antidepressant—that is, take twice as much the next day. In fact, to do so may bring on its side effects; for example, one may be very sleepy the next day. Again, because the pace of build up and removal is so slow, even a whole missed dose won't make a big difference to the level in the body.

Most people can take 600 or even 900 milligrams of lithium at a time, so many can take their whole dose on a twice-a-day schedule, and some can even take it all at once. Lithium can be irritating to the gastrointestinal tract, however, so taking it after meals is a good idea. Lithium is handled more quickly by the body, so it is a good idea to make up any missed doses.

Don't forget that the pharmacist is an expert on medication too. If a question comes up, the odds are the pharmacist can answer it.

The last point is about blood levels. Remember that the amount of medication in the bloodstream rises after one takes a pill or capsule and then falls off until the next dose. It is important that a blood sample for a medication level be taken about twelve hours after the last dose. With lithium this usually means not taking one's morning dose the day of the test until after the blood has been drawn.

Suicide

Mood disorders are potentially fatal illnesses. Self-destructive thoughts and impulses and even suicide attempts are not uncommon in persons suffering from these illnesses. The intensely sad and oppressive feelings these illnesses cause can make life itself seem a difficult, even overwhelming burden and an unwanted thing. Minimizing the risk of self-destructive behavior is a necessary part of living with a mood disorder and needs to be discussed in detail.

Perhaps the most effective means of minimizing the risk for suicide is the prevention of episodes of illness. This may seem so obvious as to not bear discussion, yet, as with many ideas that may seem obvious, it is a rather profound truth. Relapse prevention is really suicide prevention, and I invite you to reread the preceding sections dealing with relapse with this idea in mind. Persons with mood disorders should know well all the signs and symptoms of relapse and not hesitate to get in touch with the doctor should they notice these changes. The best preventative action of all in dealing with suicide is to prevent relapse.

Nevertheless, despite the best efforts of all involved, relapses do occur and the symptoms of a recurrent depression may include suicidal thoughts. The appearance of self-destructive thoughts and impulses is in itself very frightening, both to the patient and to those around him. For many centuries, tremendous stigma and disgrace has been associated with suicide, and this sense of shamefulness still makes some people reluctant to discuss these thoughts when they occur. These ideas, similar to the common misconception that "only crazy people kill themselves," only complicate what is really a simple clinical issue: suicidal thoughts and behavior are a complication of a medical illness, a serious complication that warrants immediate medical attention. For this reason, involvement of a mental health professional to assess the situation and make recommendations is a necessary and very appropriate first step.

Another common misconception about suicide is that asking a person if they are thinking of harming themselves will "plant the idea" and may thus increase the chances of suicide. There is no scientific evidence to support this idea, indeed, many persons who are having suicidal feelings are relieved to be able to talk about them.

Prediction of suicide is very difficult, but one feeling that seems to be associated with suicide attempts is hopelessness. Depressed people who express hopelessness, believe there is "no way out," or feel trapped may be at high risk of self-injurious behavior. Those close to the patient with depression need to become familiar and comfortable with words they can use to ask about suicide: "Are you bothered by feelings that life isn't worth living?" "Are you having thoughts about hurting yourself?" If there is even a hint that the answer may be yes, professional assessment of the situation is necessary. Avoiding the subject may cause the afflicted person to conceal self-destructive thoughts and feelings until they feel overwhelmed and then act on them suddenly.

To reiterate, mental health professionals know how to assess the risk and what steps to take: change of medication, dosage increase, more frequent therapy visits, hospitalization—there are many options. As I said earlier, discussing these thoughts with a professional trained in the assessment of the potentially self-destructive person can be very encouraging and reassuring for everyone involved and may in itself resolve the situation.

I want to emphasize that the professional can help best in making treatment decisions. If a member of the family with a history of heart problems suddenly developed chest pain, the family wouldn't try to decide whether or not to change medication or hospitalize—the doctor would be called immediately! The appearance of suicidal thoughts should be treated in the same way—it is a serious symptom, its appearance calls for cool heads and a contingency plan. Everyone should know who to call and not hesitate to do so.

Every year or so I will see a patient in my office who is depressed and after reassuring myself during the interview that the risk of suicide is low send them home only to get a panicked phone call from a spouse or parent, "Why didn't you put her in the hospital? Didn't she tell you she had asked me where she could buy a gun?" Contrary to popular belief, psychiatrists cannot read minds! Suicidal thoughts may be accompanied by feelings of shame, or felt by the patient to indicate weakness or being "really far gone" and so might be concealed. It's important to remember that just as there are things a person will tell their therapist and not their family, the converse is true as well. Also, suicidal thoughts, like the mood itself in depression can change throughout the day, be present on some days and not on others, or at some times of day and not others. All these factors may contribute to the patient not revealing these thoughts to the doctor. The family should not assume that the doctor will figure out in a brief interview everything that they have been observing for weeks or even months. Another key in suicide prevention is free communication—patient, family, and psychiatrist all need to be talking to each other.

Ironically, the period when persons are getting better from their depression is often a time when they are more vulnerable to suicide. Sometimes severely depressed persons are so lethargic that *any* action is too much of an effort. It is when they are getting a bit better and begin to have more energy that can be quite a dangerous time.

In the next section I will discuss involuntary treatment. When someone is suicidal or even possibly suicidal, one should not hesitate to invoke the legal procedures available to get a person the help they need.

Here are a few very simple and practical recommendations that will reduce the risk of suicide and that need to be exercised every day, in advance, in a household in which a mood disorder person resides, not just during a crisis:

I have already mentioned that it is important for persons with mood disorders to avoid alcohol. Abstinence becomes even more critical if depression has set in and is essential if suicidal feelings develop. Alcohol is disinhibiting, that is, it causes people to lose their inhibitions and become more impulsive. It's not difficult to see how dangerous this is in the depressed person. A significant percentage of persons who commit suicide are intoxicated when they do so; alcohol should be scrupulously avoided by depressed persons.

Suicide prevention measures also include throwing out old and leftover medications and asking family members to keep the pill bottles of current medications.

Persons with mood disorders who have access to firearms must seriously examine their need for such access. There are some studies that indicate that in states where there are more strict gun control laws, there are lower suicide rates: what is true in a population as a whole probably has application in the case of the individual. Is the risk of access to a highly lethal means of self-destruction justifiable for a person at greater risk of suicide than the average person? The answer seems obvious to me: persons with mood disorders should not have guns in the house—ever.

Suicidal persons are almost always ambivalent; they do not want to die but feel they have little choice or option. Patients with mood disorders need to recognize that when the light at the end of the tunnel seems to fade out that this itself is a symptom of their disease, not something to be acted on. Even though mood disorders do not often cause the affected person to lose touch with reality, reality is certainly colored by the mood state—an abnormal state— and reality is distorted.

When I was in the third grade, I flunked an eye exam at school and was taken off to the optometrist to get glasses. I'll never forget the first time I wore them. I was astonished at the clarity and brilliance of objects as ordinary as street signs and fire hydrants and was quite jolted to realize that my view of the world had been so dim and foggy without my even knowing it. Perception is reality. The depressed individual must not make judgments about the heaviness of his burden in life; his perception, his reality is distorted, fuzzy, and inaccurate. The pessimism and hopelessness he feels are the hallmarks of illness; they are symptoms to be treated, not true feelings to be acted upon. At the risk of sounding flippant, I want to quote something a colleague once said to me: "Suicide is a permanent solution to a *temporary* problem." Perhaps this should be the guiding principle and motto in suicide prevention.

The Family

The problems and challenges of recovery and the control of mood disorder affect the entire family. Since the illness can be lifelong, one person's problems can affect several generations.

The first task each family member must accomplish is to *understand*. There are so many misconceptions and myths about psychiatric illness, psychiatry, and psychiatric medication that seem ingrained in American thinking (see "Stigma" below) that those with mood disorders need all the support and allies they can get in their battle with illness. What patients do not need is someone telling them to "shape up" or "snap out of it." The most destructive and cruel thing one can do is to criticize them for being weak or lazy or for having "no willpower."

Perhaps the most important role for family members is to guide the patient into proper treatment. In mood disorders, the affected person often resists treatment; in fact resistance can be part of the illness.

HOW TO HELP WITH DEPRESSION

"My husband tells me I enjoy being depressed," a patient once told me. Can any more ridiculous statement be imagined? As I'm sure you have come to appreciate by now, the words *depressed* and *enjoy* are almost mutually exclusive. Depressed people can be unmotivated, lethargic, or perhaps irritable and complaining. They will be pessimistic and self-blaming and thus tend to reject the idea that

any treatment will help. Depression makes people avoid social contact, and this too may make getting them to accept treatment difficult. "What can a doctor do?" is a common question. Those unfamiliar
with the medical basis of depression can often see little point in
seeing a doctor for a problem with their feelings.

Sometimes this resistance is so frustrating that family members
are tempted to give in to the patient's lack of interest in treatment.
"You can't help someone who doesn't want help, can you?" Yes you
can! The very important point here is that mood disorders can crip-
ple a vital aspect of the healing process: *the anticipation of getting
well.* With this temporary disability, the depressed person is severely
handicapped in the ability to seek and continue in treatment. Since
a symptom of the illness is almost always some degree of hopelessness, expending energy in the pursuit of getting well seems a waste
of time, even a cruel joke.

This is where family and friends come in. *They* must be the
source of support and optimism in treatment. When patients say
that the medication is not helping and that there's no use in taking
it, the spouse, parent, child—whoever—needs to insist they keep
on and must not get caught up in the tendency to avoid treatment.
Depressed persons sometimes seem to be trying to make others as
pessimistic as they are. I sometimes tell family members who wonder why their relative is so complaining and rejecting that "it's the
illness talking." This is an important concept to remember. It's important not to listen too closely to such talk. It's also important
to remember that this attitude will disappear when the illness is
successfully treated.

Most of all, one must never blame the patient or be critical
of uncooperativeness. It is crucial to remember that this pessimism
and resistance are symptomatic of the illness. To criticize the depressed person for resisting treatment is like blaming someone with
a broken leg for not being able to walk. I hope that by now I need
not even mention that the symptoms of major depression (and the
other mood disorders, for that matter) are beyond the patient's ability to control and that blaming the victim of the disease is very
wrong.

On the other hand, one must not let the depressed person remain too passive, and sometimes firmness is necessary. It may seem
cruel to make depressed people get out of bed and go to a doctor's

appointment when they complain of feeling so bad, but it's the only way for them to get better.

A phrase I've come to use a lot to counter pessimism and resistance is "I'm confident."

"I know you don't feel a lot better yet, but I've noticed some improvement, and I'm confident you'll feel better soon."

"The doctor has started this medication, and I'm confident of his ability to help, so I'm going to remind you to take it every day."

"I know you don't feel like going shopping, but the doctor said you should be doing as many normal things as possible. I'm confident you'll feel better once we get there."

To feel confident, family members must be armed with knowledge about the illness and work in conjunction with the treating physician to bring about recovery. The spouse or another family member (one person should be appointed in larger families) should accompany the patient to appointments and should be in the office during at least part of the visit; the doctor will appreciate having an objective observer reporting. Remember, the patient's reports will always be colored by the symptoms of the illness, and objective information about improvement or lack of improvement is vital in making treatment decisions. There is little guidance available from the clinical laboratory or radiology department in making these decisions; only observations will help. The family can be the doctor's eyes and ears in the home and provide valuable information.

Many family members ask how much to expect from people recovering from depression. Should they go to work, to school? Basically, I encourage depressed patients to do as many normal things as they possibly can, even if they must force themselves. Though they may lack the motivation to attend to regular duties, when they do complete them they often feel a bit better for having done so. This is a good rule of thumb: *Try to do as much of what you normally do as you possibly can.* Family members should also encourage this.

On the other hand, it does no good to force too much, and relatives shouldn't nag or badger the patient. Remember that depressed people are feeling guilty enough from their illness; feeling that they are failing their families too will only add to their distress. They should be encouraged to do those things they can do successfully, especially diverting and physically stimulating activities like exercise, shopping, or gardening. On the other hand, they should be encouraged to stop trying to attend to tasks they aren't doing well; failing to succeed at school or work will only add to feelings of guilt and worthlessness.

HOW TO HELP WITH THE MANIC STATE

The family's role in helping a person who is becoming manic can be very trying, even painful, but it is extremely important. The terrible dilemma with this mental state is that patients can feel very *good*. More often they feel irritable and angry. In either case, sometimes they absolutely refuse any kind of help. Just as depression colors one's vision of the world so that help seems useless, mania can make help seem unnecessary or even threatening. As I hope I made clear earlier, mania can be a dangerous condition (see chapter 4), and early intervention is very important.

Psychiatry, the law, and authorities such as the police recognize this problem and provide legal mechanisms to get impaired people the treatment they require even when their symptoms blind them to their need for it. Every state has laws allowing those who are suffering from a psychiatric condition and showing severe symptoms to be evaluated for treatment, against their will if necessary. Sometimes invoking these laws is the only way to get a manic person into treatment. Several sources of information are available about these laws and the procedure for getting someone into treatment. Probably the best source is the local community mental health center, because the staff frequently performs such evaluations. General hospital emergency room staff members also will be familiar with the procedure.

Often a family member must visit the local city hall, courthouse, or police station and give information directly to a magistrate or judge. If on hearing the information the official agrees that a psychiatric evaluation is warranted, an order of some kind will be executed allowing the police or sheriff to transport the patient to the community mental health center, an emergency room, or a psychiatric unit, depending on local procedures. Often police or deputies have special training in dealing with psychiatric patients, and occasionally they will be accompanied by mental health workers in picking up an ill person. The appearance of these authority figures itself frequently has a calming effect on even the most agitated patients, and people often become much more accepting of the need to get help.

This initial procedure, which allows the authorities to act on the word of family or friends and bring people for evaluation, usually allows only that—an evaluation—and has a short time limit, usually less than forty-eight hours. During this time patients must be examined by a physician, sometimes two physicians, and must be found to meet certain criteria for continued treatment against their will. The criteria vary from state to state but usually include finding that patients suffer from a psychiatric condition requiring treatment and that without treatment they may deteriorate, be violent or suicidal, or otherwise show impaired judgment. A doctor or several doctors can determine that these criteria are met and admit the patient to a hospital. It is essential that a family member talk to the doctor making the evaluation, because direct and objective information must be recorded about the patient's behavior that indicates the need for treatment. Patients who want to avoid treatment can sometimes "pull themselves together" for the doctor, and family members who think the symptoms and need for treatment are so obvious that they need not accompany their relatives to the evaluation may find them back on the doorstep in a few hours!

After the physician admits the patient, there is always a hearing by a magistrate, judge, or hearing officer, usually a few days after the admission. This hearing determines that the involuntary admission was proper and legal and that the patient does indeed meet criteria for involuntary hospitalization. This is usually done in the hospital, often in a conference room with only a few people present. Although it is a legal proceeding, it is not a big courtroom scene; rather it is private, often informal, and there is an effort not to intimidate anyone.

It is important to remember that involuntary treatment involves curtailing a person's freedom and that the law takes it very seriously. There are safeguards to prevent the abuse of these laws, which in some countries have made a mockery of psychiatry and medicine when innocent people with "sick" political views are imprisoned in so-called hospitals. Often the patients either are assigned an attorney or are allowed to bring their own advocate. Again, it is important that the family be present so that the facts about the person's illness and symptoms can be presented directly by objective observers. If it is clear that treatment is needed to avoid a dangerous situation, the person will be committed to the hospital for a limited period. The doctor can always discharge the patient sooner, but if hospitalization is still necessary at the expiration of the time limit, another hearing must be held.

In some states involuntary treatment of outpatients is possible. The procedures for this type of commitment are usually similar to those for hospitalization. Again, the local community mental health center is the best source of information about these options.

It is important to remember that the legal procedures to get a person into a hospital and into treatment do only that. The patient does not lose any other rights, and property or testamentary rights and privileges are not in any way affected.

OTHER FAMILY ISSUES

Mood disorders take a toll on the family of the affected person as well as on the patient. Living with a depressed person can be demoralizing even for those who do not suffer from the illness, and the manic state can cause great upheaval in the family. As with any other illness whose course can be long, everyone can get very tired of dealing with it. Family members need to take care of their own needs for support and encouragement to prevent getting "burned out." We clinicians can derive support from our colleagues. We go to conventions and meetings to keep up on the latest developments and see the improvements in treatment and the new discoveries that will make our work easier. Most of all, these activities allow us to reaffirm to ourselves that we are doing good work, and practicing with high standards, and that everyone has challenging patients and feels discouraged at times—that this is not a sign of lack of dedication or commitment. Family members need the same kind of support and can get it by participating in the treatment of their relative and by getting involved in organizations that have the same goals—improving the care of those with psychiatric disorders.

Mental health professionals can help with all kinds of unhappiness, and the unhappiness, frustration, and discouragement that can arise from a mood disorder in the family are no exception. Counseling and psychotherapy can deal with these issues too. In helping someone else with emotional problems, caretakers should be aware of their own emotional needs and get support when their inner resources are strained. Fortunately, there are more and more organizations that are supportive of both the patient and the family. The Mental Health Association has chapters all over the country. It was largely responsible for the reform of psychiatric care in state hospitals and now continues to serve as an advocate for those with psychiatric problems, educate the public about mental health issues, and work to reduce the stigma of psychiatric problems and treatment. The National Alliance for the Mentally Ill was started by the families of persons with psychiatric illnesses and has evolved into a powerful and effective advocacy group. AMI lobbies for wider range and greater availability of mental health services, education of the public in psychiatric issues, and reform of insurance laws to benefit those with psychiatric disorders.

A newer and extremely important organization for patients and their families to become familiar with is the National Depressive and Manic Depressive Association (call or write for information to NDMDA, Merchandise Mart, Box 3395, Chicago, IL 60654; (312) 939-2442). This relatively new organization aims to promote research on mood disorders, combat stigma, advocate change in the law and public mental health policies, and most of all, provide information, support, and encouragement to mood disorder patients and their families. NDMDA already has many local chapters that run support groups and educational sessions for those with mood disorders. It will send a current list of its chapters as well as other local groups that provide services to patients with mood disorders and their families. Its newsletter has information about new treatments. The association provides reading lists and has a large list of publications that can be ordered from NDMDA by mail. In addition, it sponsors conventions and workshops. (They sent me a "Honk If You're on Lithium" bumper sticker when I called to ask for information!)

By scanning local newspapers or asking the local chapter of the Mental Health Association, you can obtain information about all these groups as well as about educational meetings and lectures put on by hospitals, medical schools, and community mental health centers. Community mental health centers often have a board of directors or a community advisory board. Through membership on such boards, those affected by mood disorders can have a very direct voice in the development of services and the structure and activities of these provider agencies.

To reiterate what I said earlier, information and knowledge are our most powerful weapons against mood disorders.

Psychotherapy

What role does psychotherapy play in the treatment of mood disorders? Before I try to answer this question, it might be useful to talk for a moment about what psychotherapy is. Psychotherapy, defined as simply as possible, is the treatment of emotional problems by psychological means—"talk" therapy. Counseling, concerned listening, objective advice, education—all these ways of helping can be broadly considered psychotherapy. Psychotherapists all have their own definitions of psychotherapy, and the definitions may vary quite a bit, but I think most of them will agree that psychotherapy is the process of helping people feel better by understanding themselves and learning new approaches to life's problems. Because of psychotherapy's emphasis on the interplay between inner mental experiences, memories, emotions, logic, conscience, and so forth, the point of view or therapeutic orientation of the psychotherapist is also called the *dynamic* approach to psychiatry.

Counseling is a rather direct form of therapy that essentially consists of giving advice. A therapist who tends to give advice or make recommendations is also said to be practicing a directive form of therapy. Many therapists are taught that giving advice is not therapeutic, because the patient usually has already sought advice from others and knows the path to improvement but lacks the confidence to do the right things to feel better.

Psychotherapy based on the principles of Freud emphasizes the past, especially childhood, and teaches that traumatic or merely difficult experiences in early life can poison many later experiences and relationships because these forgotten traumas linger unresolved in the unconscious mind. Freudian or psychoanalytic therapy emphasizes that patients bring these unconscious memories to every new relationship, including that with the therapist, and that if the therapists are very passive, not injecting any of their own personality into the therapeutic encounter, these memories will cause patients to replay in the therapeutic relationship the problems, fears, false hopes, and unrealistic expectations that cause them to have problems in life. In the most intensive form of Freudian psychotherapy, psychoanalysis, the therapist does not even face the patient but sits out of sight while the patient lies comfortably on a couch, able to concentrate totally on thoughts and feelings. The therapist helps identify psychological problems as rooted in the past so that the patient can discover, learn to recognize, and get rid of this "emotional baggage."

Most psychotherapy contains elements of both the directive, advice-giving counseling style and also the more passive, analytic style of letting patients do the talking while the therapist points out inconsistent or illogical problem-solving attempts that they must correct from their own inner resources. There are as many styles of therapy as there are therapists. These few paragraphs barely scratch the surface, but I think even this briefest of introductions indicates that whatever the style of psychotherapy, directive or analytical, it is an approach to helping patients that is very different from prescribing medication.

It is important to remember that for many years psychotherapy was practically the only approach available for helping persons with mood disorders, and that the biological concepts we now discuss in explaining mood disorders are comparatively recent. As biological theory and interventions such as medication and ECT were developed, there tended to be a division among psychiatrists about the comparative value placed on biological intervention (medication) and psychological intervention (psychotherapy). Psychiatrists considered themselves biologically oriented or dynamically oriented, but usually not both. In fact, not too long ago there was still a bit of name calling between the two camps. The biologically oriented were said to be "pill pushers" who wrote perscriptions and didn't talk to their patients, and the dynamically oriented were "fuzzy-thinking" wimps who held "touchy-feely" sessions instead of being "real doctors." Fortunately this silly and certainly unproductive polarity has lessened, and few psychiatrists even talk about "therapeutic orientation" any more. Any psychiatrist who is too

critical of either the biological or the dynamic orientation is one
to steer clear of!

The role psychotherapy plays in treating mood problems depends on the cause of the mood problem, and again I'm thinking
especially of depression here. As we have seen, in some cases of
depression, antidepressants will not be effective in alleviating the
symptoms (although symptomatic treatments, such as sleep medications may be helpful). Since a psychotherapist does not necessarily have to be an M.D., a nonphysician such as a psychologist, pastoral
counselor, or other professional can treat the problem effectively.

When the problem is major depression, however, a doctor clearly
needs to be in charge of the treatment, because medication is crucial. When the sufferer is in the midst of a depression, psychotherapy
broadly defined is definitely part of the treatment, but intensive
psychotherapy with a goal of helping patients understand themselves and change their approach to life will not help—in fact it
may make things worse by putting too much responsibility for getting well on the patient.

Most patients with major depression or bipolar disorder are
reassured when I tell them that they have a medical problem and
that medication will make them better, but occasionally, patients
react to this explanation as if I were not taking their problems
seriously. They want to talk about the issues that are on their minds,
their guilty feelings, their perceived failures and inadequacies. It
is important to realize that these issues are often a by-product of
the depression and not the cause of it. Psychotherapy with depressed
persons who have major depression consists of encouragement, support, education—not trying to get them to understand themselves
better. I want to emphasize, however, that this support and encouragement are nonetheless very important parts of treatment.

Another issue to mention in discussing "talking therapy" is that
sometimes a lot of talking is necessary to figure out just what kind
of therapy should be more important and what combination of
medication and psychotherapy is needed. If you'll turn back to
chapter 2 and review the case of Patty, you'll see what I mean. Patty
was the teenager who seemed to have major depression but turned
out to be going through some difficult adolescent problems. Her
depression was actually a reaction to external events, not a neu-

rotransmitter problem. Had I simply given Patty a prescription for antidepressants and sent her on her way, she might have been unhappy much longer. The opposite case, a major depression that seemed to be reactive, is illustrated in chapter 3 with the case of Alice. In both these cases several sessions, several hours of talking, were necessary to reach the deeper level of understanding necessary to make the proper diagnosis of the problem.

Because a person has major depression does not mean that more traditional psychotherapy won't be useful at some point, however. In some cases, as the person's mood gets better the "therapy" issues seem to evaporate and it becomes clear that psychotherapy is not necessary. Often, however, even as a person's mood improves, it becomes clear that psychotherapy will be useful. Exploring one's life history and reflecting on inadequate approaches to life problems are inevitable when one talks about one's feelings for a few hours and has time between sessions to think about them, and this often leads one to want to learn more about oneself and use this knowledge to adopt new coping strategies. This is the kind of process and goals accomplished in psychotherapy.

In the section on relapse, I mentioned the importance of regularizing life and cutting down on stress as a way to lessen the chances of additional episodes of these illnesses; psychotherapy can be a very important aspect of this. As we saw in the chapter on the heredity of mood disorders, these illnesses run in families, and a person who grew up in a family disrupted by the illness of a parent or another family member can carry many emotional scars into adulthood. As we have also seen, alcoholism can be associated with these illnesses, and those from homes where there was an alcohol problem are now known to frequently require psychotherapy to deal with their difficult childhoods and disrupted emotional maturation. Of course, living from day to day with a mood disorder can often be, to say the least, a difficult task. If the illness is not diagnosed until several episodes have occurred, the consequences of manic behavior or depression can cause problems in one's career, one's relationships, and many other important areas of life. In people who are suffering with a mood disorder, past and present can seem to conspire to cause tribulation and distress even when the disorder itself is in remission. When this distress builds up, it may itself make an episode of illness more likely; the treatment for these sorts of problems is psychotherapy, and thus in many instances it needs to be part and parcel of the treatment of mood disorders.

There are several new forms of psychotherapy that seem to be especially helpful in the treatment of depression, the most important being cognitive therapy. The person most closely associated with this form of psychotherapy is Dr. Aaron Beck who, along with several collaborators, has written many books and articles on depression and its treatment by cognitive therapy.

In contrast to the more traditional passive role of the psychotherapist, the practitioner of cognitive therapy is quite active, asking questions, interrupting the patient, giving directions and even assigning homework. Treatment focuses on current problems—here and now—and does not analyze the past in much detail.

The basic premise of this treatment is that persons with depression usually have attitudes or assumptions about the world and themselves (each assumption is called a schema) that can lead to negative thoughts, which in turn lead to depression. For example, suppose a young man's approach to life is dominated by the schema "You can achieve anything if you work hard enough." While there's some truth to this motto, it's not always true. Hard work might get you a promotion but you can't make the prettiest girl in the office fall in love with you just by working at it. If every time something doesn't go well in his life, this young man blames himself for being lazy, he will indeed be chronically depressed.

This theory of depression proposes that depressed persons view themselves as somehow inadequate or defective and that they tend to attribute any disappointment or unpleasant experience to this supposed defect in themselves. This view leads to automatic thoughts like "I can't do anything right" whenever a problem comes up. A young woman burns dinner and the thought "I can't do anything right" pops into her head (despite the fact that she has cooked perfect dinners every night for weeks and weeks). The patient berates herself for every failure and never takes credit for (or even takes notice of) her successes. A vicious cycle of negative thoughts and depressed feelings begins.

Cognitive therapy tries to get patients to recognize their negative automatic thoughts (negative cognitions) and see the distortions caused by their erroneous schemata. The connections between these thoughts and depressed feelings are identified and the patient is helped to replace negative thoughts with positive, reality-based thoughts and eventually to change their distorted view of themselves. (The young woman would replace "I can't do anything right" with something like "I make mistakes occasionally, but I'm basically a pretty competent person.")

Although some studies indicate that cognitive therapy can be as effective as medication in some patients, whether or not it can substitute for medical treatments is a subject of much disagreement. It is quite a specialized technique that requires special training and thus is usually available only at university medical schools and other large medical centers. Nevertheless, this technique seems to offer benefit above and beyond traditional psychotherapy in the treatment of depression and is a welcome addition to the armamentarium of available treatment options for depression.

Neither psychiatrists nor patients should close their minds to either the biological approach to helping mood disorders or the psychological. A combination of both is almost always the best way to quicker recovery.

Psychiatric Hospitalization

"Ruth certainly needs some help, but she doesn't need to be *here*." "Here" was the psychiatric unit of the finest general hospital in town. It was only two years old, staffed by expert psychiatric nurses, social workers with mental health backgrounds, occupational therapists, and other professionals. There was no lock on the door; the separate cafeteria and dining room for patients in an adjacent wing were also used by the hospital to provide dinner when the board of trustees met. The decor was beautiful and pleasant, like the dormitory of an expensive school or perhaps the executive conference and retreat center of a big corporation.

Ruth's family doctor was almost frantic on the phone that morning. "You must see this patient *today*. I've been trying to get her to see you for weeks because I haven't been able to get her depressive symptoms under control, but she's kept putting it off. Two of her friends brought her in today because she isn't sleeping, hasn't eaten in two days, and can't stop crying."

When I saw Ruth she was distraught and could hardly speak

without bursting into tears. She had small children at home and felt overwhelmed by the demands of their care. Her husband was out of town at a business meeting, and she was terrified of being alone. Her friends had been up all night trying to soothe and calm her. I agreed with her family doctor that she was having a major depressive episode.

"I want to admit you to Memorial Hospital; I think it would be best for you to be someplace where someone can take care of you, where you won't have to worry about cooking and such and can get away from the phone. I want to be a bit more aggressive with medications for depression, and this means you might be a bit sedated at first. In the hospital there'll be nurses to check your blood pressure and so forth; they know these medications and can be on the lookout for any side effects or other problems. We can change the treatment plan daily or even hourly if need be."

"Whatever you think is best," was her feeble reply. She was exhausted.

I called the hospital, and there was an empty bed. I sent Ruth home with her friends to get some clothes and toiletries and told them I would meet them at the hospital that afternoon.

When I got to the hospital to write admission orders and get Ruth's treatment started, I was surprised to find her and her friends in the visitor's waiting room. Her bags at her side, she looked as if she was ready to leave rather than to be admitted.

"Doctor, I'm frightened. I don't know if this is the right thing to do. I don't know if this is the right place for me."

"Of course you feel frightened," I said. "No one likes to be in the hospital, and besides, depression makes people feel frightened and uneasy about everything. You'll be in good hands here." I looked to her friends to support me.

I was flabbergasted at one friend's reply: "Couldn't you just give her some sleeping pills and see her as an outpatient?"

I thought to myself, "With friends like you, who needs enemies?" (Psychiatrists probably do more tongue biting than any other medical specialists.)

"Wouldn't it be better for me to be home with my family, in my own house? I don't feel very relaxed in the hospital; I'm not sure I could sleep."

"You told me you were up all last night. I don't think tonight would be much better even with sleeping pills. If being at home with your family was what you needed, you'd be feeling better by now. This is the best psychiatric unit in the city, and we were lucky to get you a bed today. Usually there's a waiting list of several days."

"I don't know what to do."

"Of course you don't; depression makes people indecisive and unsure of themselves. That's why you came to see me—right? Because you don't know how to help yourself and need expert advice. I think you will get better much more quickly in the hospital. I'll be able to be more aggressive with medication doses here." I found I was repeating myself.

"Couldn't I be on a regular medical floor? You could see me every day there."

"Medical floors are noisy and upsetting even for someone who is not depressed. The staff here is experienced in helping with depression. They know how to care for people with symptoms like being frightened, being anxious. They know the best way to help. On a medical floor the staff will give you your medication, but they won't be available to talk or be very reassuring; they're too busy. Also, you need to learn about depression and medication for depression, and your family will want to be involved in your recovery. We have special meetings for family members here to help everyone learn about depression and its treatment."

"Won't it be depressing for me to be around other depressed people or people with worse problems?"

"Most people find it's comforting to know that others have the same kind of problems, and seeing that you're not the sickest person in the hospital can be a comfort too."

Ruth finally listened to the person she was paying for expert advice—me—and admitted herself to the hospital. As I expected, she was soon home again and feeling much better.

Just as people still have all kinds of misconceptions about psychiatrists, they have misconceptions about psychiatric hospitalization. Many of these misconceptions are based on some unfortunate facts about psychiatric treatment in the distant past. You've heard the horror stories and seen the old movies, so I won't

repeat those facts except to say that in the days when there was
essentially no effective medical treatment for any psychiatric problem, many, many persons with psychiatric illnesses received inadequate care, under poor conditions, in understaffed, poorly funded
state hospitals. Fortunately those days are over. There are no more
"snake pits."

What are modern psychiatric hospitals, and psychiatric units
in general hospitals, like? Since people with psychiatric illnesses
are not usually physically incapacitated or "sick" in a physical sense,
psychiatric hospitals, or psychiatric units of general hospitals, are
a bit different from medical or surgical units. Patients wear regular
clothes, not pajamas or nightgowns, and do not spend much time
in their rooms. Psychiatric units are often laid out much like a school
dormitory, with bedrooms, a large sitting area or common area,
and perhaps some lounges in addition to the usual nursing station
and other staff areas. Patients usually eat together in a dining area.
They are often responsible for getting their own medication from
the nursing station rather than lying in bed and having it brought
to them.

There are almost always several group meetings each week,
where patients are encouraged to discuss the symptoms that brought
them into the hospital. Staff members lead these groups and help
people share and learn from one another. Because chemical depend-
ence complicates so many psychiatric problems, AA meetings or
other meetings on this subject are sometimes held on the unit.

Besides the doctor, who leads the treatment team and is ul-
timately responsible for treatment, there are many other staff
members who help in the recovery process. Social workers, who
usually have special training in working with families, often meet
with family members to gather information that will help the doctor
educate both patient and family about the treatment. They also can
help patients make practical arrangements during and after the
hospitalization, such as planning treatment after discharge, finding
child care, coordinating transportation home, and coping with insurance and Social Security issues. They often do family therapy
or marriage counseling as well, if the psychiatrist requests it. Almost
all units provide some diversions too. Patients who are depressed
often feel like just lying around or restlessly pacing the floor. A
physical therapist is often on the staff, and exercise is encouraged—

perhaps stretching exercises and calisthenics once a day—to stimulate appetite and promote sleep. Many hospitals have exercise rooms, even gymnasiums and pools. Occupational therapists provide opportunity for more focused activities, often "arts and crafts." Especially in depression, people tend to be inwardly focused and preoccupied, and a simple project like potting some seedlings or painting a figurine can help them think about something besides their bad feelings for a time and let them experience the little victory of accomplishing something and seeing the results. Also, occupational therapy provides the doctor with a valuable tool for assessing progress. It gives trained staff an opportunity to observe and measure improvement (or lack thereof) of problems such as impaired concentration, restlessness in depression or motor agitation in mania, impaired self-confidence, or irritability.

We must not forget the psychiatric nurses, for they are the glue that holds a good program together. Nurses encourage, nurture, support, and comfort their patients and answer their questions, and they record all kinds of information for the psychiatrist, from blood pressure and weight to how many hours of sleep a patient had. Good nurses don't just follow orders; they ask the doctor questions and make suggestions. Many hospitals have a "primary nurse" system where one nurse is assigned to coordinate care throughout the patient's stay and be a consistent contact between the patient and the rest of the staff.

What kinds of psychiatric problems call for hospitalization? Just as with any other medical problem, the hospital is necessary when symptoms are so severe that people's ability to care for themselves and their families is disrupted, when they need speedy assessment and diagnosis because of rapid appearance of or change in their symptoms, or when an intensity of treatment is warranted that is not possible in an outpatient setting. In earlier chapters I described some of the more serious symptoms of mood disorders—delusions, very high activity level, and agitation. These symptoms require hospitalization. Sometimes hospitalization is a good idea to *prevent* these symptoms. ECT requires hospitalization (though some hospitals will allow outpatient ECT if the patient will have plenty of care and supervision at home).

Hospitalization simply speeds up the process of recovery. Instead of taking several weeks to get to know a patient, with the help of a good staff I can make a much better assessment in a day or two. In the hospital, staff members can objectively measure how much the patient is sleeping or eating, and progress is assessed daily by professionals. Treatments, especially medications that are not working, can be changed immediately. Problems can be more easily treated before they become too severe. When a person starts on lithium or antidepressants, blood tests can be done daily if necessary, so the therapeutic dose can be reached quickly. Side effects can be monitored and treated at once.

Naturally, if the patient is having suicidal thoughts hospitalization is necessary. Also, as sometimes happens in the manic state, patients who are having aggressive feelings can be helped to control their impulses much better in the hospital. Hospitalization is a good idea if the symptoms are severe or if the patient is in danger of deteriorating—in any situation where time is of the essence. I hesitate to hospitalize patients who can still manage to go to work or school, but if they are not able to carry out these activities, that in itself makes hospitalization a good resource.

Do freestanding psychiatric hospitals have advantages over psychiatric units in general hospitals? I think there are advantages and disadvantages to each. The general hospital with a good psychiatric program may be the first choice for those whose health is frail, perhaps because they have been depressed for a long time and are malnourished or dehydrated, because they are elderly, or because they have another illness. The general hospital has more medical support—laboratories, an X-ray department, a large medical staff with many specialities, and so forth.

The advantage of freestanding psychiatric hospitals perhaps is their very lack of the "medical" quality. They tend to be smaller and often have more amenities such as a large cafeteria, exercise rooms, meeting rooms, and occupational therapy rooms. These are the hospitals that may have tennis courts and swimming pools.

Perhaps the best of both worlds can be found in the university medical center. Because these hospitals are large, they also have large units devoted to psychiatry and so may have the amenities and physical facilities of the freestanding hospitals and also the range of medical support of the general hospital. That they are part of a medical school means the latest in treatment is often accessible, perhaps including new medications not available to other hospitals. In difficult cases of mood disorders, a trip to a different part of the state or even out of state may be well worth the effort.

Sometimes my patients come to the hospital thinking they will be put to bed and left alone to "rest." One patient asked me, "Isn't there a hospital where I don't have to participate in all these activities?" "There is," I replied, "but I don't admit my patients there unless there are no other beds available in town." Good psychiatric programs encourage, even insist on, activity not passivity, socialization not withdrawal, and active sharing, learning, and helping each other, especially in group settings, rather than isolation. They promote wellness and recovery by pushing patients to be as independent and as responsible for their recovery as possible.

Stigma

Unfortunately, there still is stigma attached to any type of psychiatric disorder, and mood disorders are no exception. One patient of mine had been doing extremely well on lithium for some months after having been ill for nearly a year because she had been incorrectly diagnosed. She told me she was becoming serious about a young man. "When and how do I tell him I take medication to keep my mood stable?" I had no easy answer for her. "What do I tell people when they ask me why I was in the hospital?" patients often ask. Again, I know of no easy answer.

I suppose a good basic fact to remember is that one's medical history is very properly considered a private matter. Those who feel compelled to share every detail of their gallbladder operations with anyone who will listen probably don't realize just how boring they really are. On the other hand, people who probe even brief acquaintances for information about what a biopsy showed, what medication they are taking, and so forth are going far beyond the boundaries of politeness and good taste and should simply be told that those are personal matters that bear no discussion. Medical records are strictly confidential and cannot be released to anyone without the patient's permission. Some states require special kinds of permission for release of psychiatric records.

Close friends and family will understand about a mood dis-

order, though they may need a little educating. A trusted friend
or co-worker, someone that you would feel comfortable discussing
any other serious medical matter with and who is in a position
to help and support, will be able to handle a mood disorder just
as well as any other personal matter. Those who choose to pull away
or who resist education are fair-weather friends you are well rid
of anyway, however painful the parting.

Sometimes patients with a mood disorder ask me, "Do I have
a mental illness?" I usually tell them that they certainly have an
illness, and that since the most prominent symptoms—feelings,
thoughts, and behaviors—are in the realm of things considered
"mental" rather than "physical" as most laymen understand those
terms, "Well yes, I suppose you do." Unfortunately the term *mental
illness* has come to have all kinds of negative connotations beyond
this clumsy definition. Some of the myths are that people with mental illness are dangerous, that mental illness is incurable, and that
its victims must be locked up forever; that the symptoms of mental
illness are bizarre and shocking; that victims of mental illness, indeed their whole families, are somehow cursed or at least tainted.

I won't go through these myths and refute them one by one,
for if you have read the other chapters you know such horrors certainly do not apply to mood disorders. It is interesting to realize
that not so very long ago these very same myths were held to be
true of two other forms of "mental illness"—that is, illnesses with
behavioral symptoms—epilepsy and mental retardation. At one
time those with epilepsy were confined in state mental hospitals.
The mentally retarded were once considered physically dangerous
and aggressive as well as sexually aggressive, and therefore were
seen as needing lifelong institutional confinement to protect the
community. Education has largely removed the stigma associated
with epilepsy and mental retardation, but the connotations of
shame, dangerousness, and unpredictability remain with the term
mental illness. Therefore it is a term to be tossed out of our vo-
cabulary—put into the trash bin with *madness* and *insanity*.

Another issue I'll mention briefly is discrimination, the ugly
fruit growing from the seed of stigma. Those who feel they have
been discriminated against because of a history of mood disorder

should consult an attorney, for it is illegal to discriminate because of a particular kind of illness. Again, the NDMDA and the Mental Health Association, who make the fight against stigma a priority, are excellent resources for support and encouragement.

One form of institutionalized discrimination is only now beginning to receive attention—medical insurance coverage for psychiatric benefits. Almost all types of medical insurance, whether the traditional indemnity plans or health maintenance organizations (HMOs) and such cover psychiatric problems at a lower rate than other illnesses. The number of office visits may be limited (some plans provide no outpatient psychiatric benefits whatever), and the copayment (the amount the patient must pay toward care) is often higher. Frequently there is a strict limit on inpatient days in psychiatric units, a limit separate from other inpatient days. Although solid medical evidence has existed for years that mood disorders are medical problems just like, for example, Parkinson's disease, and though an M.D. must treat them with medicines or other medical treatments like ECT, do blood tests and so forth, these illnesses are separated from all the rest and not covered as fully by the vast majority of insurance plans. In my opinion the insurance industry has taken advantage of ignorance and stigma to evade responsibility to clients and increase profits. The organizations working to pass laws requiring "parity"—that is, insurance coverage for psychiatric problems comparable to that for other medical problems— are the Mental Health Association, the National Depressive and Manic Depressive Association, and the Alliance for the Mentally Ill.

EIGHT

SUMMING UP

I wrote this book to help fill a void in my patients' knowledge that became apparent to me as I started a general psychiatric practice away from the major university medical center where I received my training in psychiatry. What I saw was that many people who came to me for treatment, even highly educated and well-informed people—people who ran multimillion dollar businesses or were bank presidents or engineers—hadn't a clue to the medical basis of some types of depression, mood swings, and other mood disorders. Some had heard vaguely about "chemical imbalances" but were ignorant of even the basic facts of a problem they may have had for years. Compounding this ignorance were the stigma associated with psychiatric problems, mistaken notions about psychiatrists, and frightening media representations of ECT and psychiatric hospitals. It becomes clear why, although mood disorders are extremely common, many sufferers receive no treatment or inadequate treatment. I hope that I've helped break down the barriers to treatment for some and aided those already in treatment to understand their problem better.

Now that the basic facts about these disorders have been set out, let me indulge in a little speculation. In many other illnesses of the body, abnormal functioning is clearly linked to tissue destruction of one type or another. A tumor grows and presses on a nerve, and paralysis results. Remove the tumor and the function may return. The pneumococcus bacterium invades lung cells, cells die, and the lung fills up with pus and blood; but remove the invader and the lung cells regenerate. In sickle-cell anemia, abnormal hemoglobin causes blood cells to elongate and clog blood vessels; oxygen-starved tissues begin to die, and pain and dysfunction result.

What a different sort of process mood disorders seem to result from! By almost every measure, nothing seems amiss in the body, and not only medication but light therapy and sleep deprivation can help in some cases. No death of cells, no bacterial invaders, no tumors.

Scientists have started to think there must be a "mood system" in the body that allows mood to change in response to certain events and stimuli and that also returns mood to "neutral"—some "set point." Just as a temperature center in the brain returns the body temperature to 98.6° Fahrenheit by turning on sweating or shivering, the "mood center" must return the mood to neutral from depression after a disappointment, from euphoria after some happy event. Mood disorders might result from a malfunction in this center. If the set point changes, pervasive, unrelenting depression may result. Sensitivity may change so that the center overshoots in both directions in erratic patterns, resulting in cyclothymia. Perhaps in some people the center is connected too strongly to other regulators such as the biological clocks regulating sleep and the menstrual cycle, and seasonal affective disorder or premenstrual symptoms result. This type of conceptualizing makes it apparent why these disorders have remained so difficult to understand.

If one of our colonial forefathers (or more probably foremothers) woke up on a winter morning to find the house bitterly cold, she would have gone to the fireplace or Franklin stove to see what was the matter—why the fire had gone out. If she traveled through time and woke up in a modern house, a chill in the air might make her go down to the cellar and try to figure out the furnace. She'd find a heating element and a device to circulate the warm air. She might understand the mechanism very well, since it is really not so different from the heating devices she would be familiar with. She would never, however, think of checking the thermostat. The concept of an independent controlling device that senses changes in the environment and operates the furnace in response to those changes would be totally outside her experience.

Neuroscience is beginning to figure out the "thermostat." Thinking of mood disorders in this way, it's not so hard to accept that manipulating sleep and light help in these disorders; these manipulations may be resetting the mood thermostat. ECT becomes more understandable too; just as electrical energy can reset the rhythm of the stalled heart, ECT may reset the mood regulator in the brain.

Bipolar disorder is a perplexing illness at first glance. One disease that causes both depression *and* euphoria? But once again, if we begin to imagine a malfunctioning regulator rather than simply too much of this chemical or too little of that one as a cause for all the symptoms, the facts begin to make some sense.

The investigations of neurotransmitters and medication effects are leading toward an understanding of the chemical workings of mood. The discoveries about mood changes after stroke are pointing toward the location and anatomical organization of the system. Now that the conceptual leap has been made from simple cause-and-effect reasoning to cybernetics (the study of automatic control systems), working out the details is only a matter of time and technology.

In short, our understanding of mood disorders is growing at great speed, and many researchers are optimistic that better ways of detecting, diagnosing, and most important, treating these enigmatic illnesses are not far off. Identifying the genes for mood disorders may allow prenatal detection of afflicted individuals and reliable genetic counseling. Better medications will be developed as the chemistry of mood is better understood. Other treatments such as therapeutic light and sleep phase advance will become more sophisticated and reliable and may perhaps eliminate the need for medication. Special EEGs or brain scans may help in diagnosing mood disorders in the future and guide the physician on when to start and stop treatment in an individual, eliminating long periods of unnecessary treatment of a patient who is in remission and allowing us to start treatment before symptoms emerge and interfere with functioning.

In the meantime, those with symptoms of mood disorders must take advantage of the very good treatments that are available.

Stigma is no excuse for ignoring the symptoms. Families must insist that affected relatives get treatment, even if it means initiating commitment procedures. The treatments are effective and safe; the consequences of ignoring the illness can be fatal.

Involvement in organizations such as the National Depressive and Manic Depressive Association will help advance knowledge, increase research funding, educate the general public and reduce stigma, and obtain insurance parity for psychiatric disorders.

Many paths are being taken in the search for better diagnosis and treatment of mood disorders, and most stretch far beyond the horizon—no dead ends in sight. People who suffer from mood disorders can be more than just hopeful that the future will be brighter for them; they can be *confident* that it will.

FURTHER READING

Andreasen, Nancy C. *The Broken Brain*. New York: Harper and Row, 1985.

A well-written and informative survey of the development of modern psychiatry as the study of the brain as the organ of the mind.

Duke, Patty. *Call Me Anna*. New York: Bantam Books, 1987.

A famous actress writes about her battle with bipolar disorder and her victory over it.

Fieve, Ronald. *Moodswing: The Third Revolution in Psychiatry*. New York: Bantam Books, 1975.

Although a bit dated now, a vivid and engrossing account of the development of lithium treatment and of its dramatic power to treat bipolar disorder.

Klein, Nathan S. *From Sad to Glad*. New York: Putnam, 1974.

Lithium and Manic Depression: A Guide. Madison, Wisc.: Lithium Information Center, 1988.

Concise and to the point.

Papolos, Demetri F., M.D., and Janet Papolos. *Overcoming Depression*. New York: Harper and Row, 1987.

Complete and detailed discussions of mood disorders, somewhat more technical and "scientific." Extensive bibliography.

Weeks, Clair. *Hope and Help for Your Nerves.* New York: Bantam
    Books, 1969.
    Despite its date of publication, the best book ever written for
    sufferers of panic attacks. Encouraging and helpful for anyone
    with a psychiatric illness.
Wender, Paul H., and Donald F. Klein. *Mind, Mood and Medicine.*
    New York: Farrar, Straus and Girox, 1982.

The National Depressive and Manic Depressive Association has a
reading list that includes many of these books and offers a "mail-
order bookstore." Write to NDMDA, Merchandise Mart, Box 3395,
Chicago, Illinois 60654 or call (312) 939-2442.

INDEX

Acetylcholine, 9, 51, 90
Adapin, 44. *See also* Antidepressant
   medications
Addison's disease, 166
Adjustment disorder, 30-31
Adolescents: mood disorders in,
   113-15; suicide in, 116-17
Adrenal glands, 140, 166. *See also*
   Steroids, adrenal
Affective disorder: classification of,
   34-41, 86-87; definition of, 12;
   depression of (*see* Major depression)
Agoraphobia. *See* Panic attacks
Alcoholics Anonymous, 158
Alcoholism, 155, 156-63
Alcohol use, 188, 192
Allergies to medication, 51-52
Alliance for the Mentally Ill, 199, 213
Alprazolam, 150, 165. *See also*
   Anxiolytic medications
Alzheimer's disease, 111-12, 179
Amines, 55, 75-76, 90-91
Amish, 154-55
Amitriptyline, 50, 134. *See also*
   Antidepressant medications

Amphetamines: abuse of, 161-62;
   therapeutic uses, 57
Analysis. *See* Psychoanalysis
"Angel dust," 162
Anhedonia, 22
Anorexia nervosa, 125, 156
Anticholinergic side effects, 51
Anticipatory anxiety, 145
Anticonvulsant medications, 100
Antidepressant medications: history,
   43; side effects of, 49-51; treatment
   with, 45-49, 53-55, 98-99, 188-89
Antipsychotic medications, 57-60,
   99-100; side effects, 59-60
Anxiety, 26, 144-51
Anxiolytic medications, 9, 57, 150, 165
Appetite changes in mood disorders, 19,
   25, 138
Ascendin, 44. *See also* Antidepressant
   medications
Attention deficit disorder, 116
Aventyl, 44. *See also* Antidepressant
   medications

"Baby blues," 118-20
Barbiturates, 165
Beck, Aaron, 204
Behavior problems in children,
    114-15
Benzodiazepines. *See* Anxiolytic
    medications
Bereavement, 4
Biological clock. *See* Chronobiology
Bipolar depression, 86
Bipolar disorder: neurochemistry,
    90-91; symptoms, 80-86; treatment,
    92-101
Bipolar II, 89, 142
Birth control pills, 165
Blood pressure medications, 164.
    See also Reserpine
Blood tests: for affective disorder,
    75-77; for antidepressants, 53, 125,
    189; for lithium, 94-95, 189
Brain damage. *See* Stroke

Cade, John, 93
Calcium, 167-68
Cancer, 163-65, 169
Carbemazepine, 100
Carbohydrate craving, 138
Cerebrovascular accident. *See* Stroke
Chemical dependency. *See* Alcoholism;
    Drug abuse
Children: mood disorders in, 113-15;
    suicide in, 116-17
Chlorpromazine, 43, 57-58. *See also*
    Antipsychotic medications
Cholecystokinin, 134
Chromosomes, 155. *See also* Genetics
Chronic fatigue syndrome, 168-69
Chronic pain syndrome, 130-36
Chronobiology, 76-77, 136-37,
    139-42, 173
Circadian rhythm, 137
Clonazepam, 100
Cocaine, 162
Codeine. *See* Narcotics
Cognitive therapy, 204-5

Commitment. *See* Involuntary
    commitment
Community mental health centers, 184
Constipation, 25-26, 51
Cortisol, 76-77, 137, 140. *See also*
    Steroids, adrenal
Counseling. *See* Psychotherapy
Cybernetics, 216
Cyclothymia, 87-90

Darkness and mood disorders. *See*
    Seasonal affective disorder
Delusions, 72
Dementia, 111; syndrome of depression,
    108-13
Depersonalization, 145
Depression: definitions of, 3-5;
    syndrome of, 37. *See also* Dysthymia;
    Major depression
Depressive equivalent, 114
Depressive spectrum disease, 155-56
Derealization, 145
Desipramine, 50. *See also*
    Antidepressant medications
Desyrel. *See* Trazodone
Dexamethasone suppression test,
    76-77
Diazepam, 9, 150, 165. *See also*
    Anxiolytic medications
Discrimination. *See* Stigma
Diurnal variation of mood, 20, 137
Dopamine, 9, 10-11
Doxepine, 50. *See also* Antidepressant
    medications
Drug abuse, 54-55, 160-63
Dynamic psychotherapy. *See* Psycho-
    analysis; Psychotherapy
Dysthymic disorder, 40

EB virus, 168
ECT. *See* Electroconvulsive therapy
EEG, 171
Elavil. *See* Amitriptyline
Electroconvulsive therapy:
    administration technique, 62-65,

69-70; development, 61-62; side
effects, 65-66; versus medication,
74-75; treatment uses, 61, 101, 112
Electroencephalogram (EEG), 171
Endep, 44. *See also* Antidepressants
Endogenous depression. *See* Major
depression
Endorphin, 135
Epilepsy, 61, 212
Epstein-Barr virus, 168
Equanil, 165
EST. *See* Electroconvulsive therapy
Estrogens. *See* Sex steroids, female
Ethchorvynol, 165

Family: role in treatment of depression,
193-96; role in treatment of mania,
196-98; support, 198-200
Fibromyositis, 133
Fluoxetine, 50, 53. *See also*
Antidepressant medications
Freud, Sigmund. *See* Psychoanalysis

GABA, 9
Genetics: mechanism, 152-55; of mood
disorders, 126, 154-56

Hallucinations, 142-43
Headaches, 25, 132-33
Hepatitis, 168
Heredity. *See* Genetics
Heroin. *See* Narcotics
Hibernation, 139
Hormones, 166-68. *See also*
Cholecystokinin; Melatonin; Steroids,
adrenal; Sex steroids; Thyroid
hormones
Hospitals, psychiatric, 205-9
Huntington's disease (Huntington's
Chorea), 153, 168
"Hyperactivity," 56, 116
Hypersomnia, 25, 50, 138
Hyperthyroidism. *See* Thyroid hormones
Hypomania, 89, 137

Hypothalamus, 167
Hypothyroidism. *See* Thyroid hormones

Imipramine, 115. *See also*
Antidepressant medications
Imvarate, 44. *See also* Antidepressant
medications
Insomnia: in depression, 16-17, 19,
172-73; in mania, 165
Insurance, 213
Involuntary commitment, 196-98
Involutional melancholia, 21, 118
Irritable bowel syndrome, 132

Kraeplin, Emil, 137
Kuhn, Roland, 43

Lead poisoning, 166
Light therapy. *See* Phototherapy
Lithium: blood test, 94-95, 189;
development, 92-94; side effects,
95-98; therapeutic uses, 57, 92-98
Ludiomil, 44. *See also* Antidepressant
medications

Major depression: course, 20, 26;
neurochemistry, 44, 46-48; symptoms,
23-27; treatment, 42-66
Mania, 80-84; symptoms, 82; treatment,
92-101
Manic-depressive illness. *See* Bipolar
disorder
MAO inhibitors, 55-56, 147
Maprotiline, 50. *See also*
Antidepressants
Marijuana, 161
Medication, 187-98; side effects and
allergies, 51-52
Melancholia, 5
Melatonin, 139-42
Mellaril. *See* Thioridazine
Memory loss: side effect of ECT, 65-66;
symptom of depression, 111-13
Menstrual period, 120-26
Mental Health Association, 184, 199, 213

"Mental illness," 212-13
Meprobamate, 165
Methqualone, 165
Methylphenidate, 57
MHPG, 75
Miltown, 165
Mixed affective state, 85
Mononucleosis, 168
Mood: definition, 3-6; effect of ECT on,
    62-64; neurochemistry, 7, 11-14,
    44-45, 215-16
Mood swings. See Bipolar disorder;
    Cyclothymia
Morphine. See Narcotics
Multiple sclerosis, 168

Narcotics, 134-36. See also Drug abuse
Nardil, 44. See also MAO inhibitors
National Depressive and Manic
    Depressive Association, 199, 213
Negative thoughts. See Cognitive
    therapy
Nembutal, 165
Neurosis, 31
Neurotic depression, 31. See also
    Dysthymia
Neurotransmitters, 8-14; in bipolar
    disorder, 90-91; in depression, 44,
    46-48
Nightmares, 23
Norepinephrine, 9, 44, 162-64
Norpramin, 44. See also Antidepressant
    medications
Nortriptyline, 50. See also
    Antidepressant medications
Nursing, 180, 209

Obsessional thoughts, 24-25, 70
Occupational therapy, 209
Opiate receptors, 134-36
Opium. See Narcotics
Oral contraceptives, 165
Organic affective syndrome, 163-64,
    169-70

Pain, 25, 130-33
Pain medications. See Narcotics
Palpitations, 144-48
Pamelor, 44. See also Antidepressant
    medications
Panic attacks, 144-51
Paranoia, 84
Parathyroid hormones, 167
Parkinson's disease, 10-11, 168
Parnate, 44. See also MAO inhibitors
Pastoral counseling, 180
PCP, 162
Perphenazine, 60. See also
    Antipsychotic medications
Pertrofan, 44. See also Antidepressant
    medications
Phencyclidine, 162
Phenylzine, 50. See also MAO inhibitors
Photoperiod, 139
Phototherapy, 138-42
Pineal gland, 139-42
Pituitary gland, 167
Placidyl, 165
PMS. See Premenstrual syndrome
Poisons, 165-66
Postpartum depression, 118-20
Prednisone. See Steroids, adrenal
Pregnancy, 118-20, 188
Premenstrual syndrome, 120-26
Prevalence of mood disorders, 118, 154
Progesterone. See Sex steroids, female
Prozac. See Fluoxetine
Pseudo-dementia, 111
Psychiatrists, 178-79
Psychoanalysis, 182, 200-201
Psychologists, 180
Psychomotor retardation, 25
Psychosomatic, 133
Psychotherapy, 78, 200-205
Psychotic depression, 31, 71-73
Psychotic symptoms, 58. See also
    Delusions; Hallucinations

Quaalude, 165

"Rapid cycling," 99-100
Reactive depression, 27-31, 36. *See also*
    Adjustment disorder
Relapse prevention, 185-87
REM latency, 173
REM sleep, 172
Reserpine, 7-8, 164
Ritalin, 57

SAD, 136-42
Schizoaffective disorder, 143
Schizophrenia, 43, 72, 142-43
School refusal, 115
Schou, Morgans, 94
Seasonal affective disorder (SAD),
    136-42
Seconal, 165
Secondary depression, 31, 161
Sedative/hypnotic medications. *See*
    Anxiolytic medications
Sedatives; as cause of mood symptoms,
    165-66. *See also* Antipsychotic
    medications; Anxiolytic
    medications
Senility. *See* Dementia
Serotonin, 44; in chronic pain, 134.
    See also Amines
Sex drive: in depression, 19, 25;
    in mania, 83
Sex ratio of mood disorders, 118,
    125-26
Sex steroids, female, 118-23, 125-26,
    165
Sex steroids, male, 134
Shock treatments. *See* Electrocon-
    vulsive therapy
Sinequan, 44. *See also* Antidepressant
    medications
Sleep, normal, 172
Sleep architecture, 171-73
Sleep deprivation (treatment for
    depression), 172-74
Sleep disturbances. *See* Hypersomnia;
    Insomnia

Sleep phase advance, 173
Slow wave sleep, 172
Social workers, 180, 208
Steroids, adrenal, 119-20; as cause of
    mood symptoms, 73, 164-65
Stigma, 211-13
Stimulants, 57
Stroke: and depression, 126-30; and
    mania, 130
Suicide: in children and adolescents,
    116-17; complication of mood
    disorders, 189-92; prevention,
    192-93
Support groups, 198-200
SWS (slow wave sleep), 172
Synapse, 46-48
Syndrome, 32

Tegretol, 100
Testosterone, 134
Thioridazine, 58. *See also* Antipsychotic
    medications
"Third psychosis," 143
Thorazine. *See* Chlorpromazine
Thyroid hormones: as cause of mood
    symptoms, 166-67; as treatment for
    depression, 56-57
Tofranil. *See* Imipramine
Tranquilizers, major. *See* Antipsychotic
    medications
Tranquilizers, minor. *See* Anxiolytic
    medications
Tranylcypromine, 50. *See also* MAO
    inhibitors
Trazodone, 50, 134. *See also*
    Antidepressant medications
Tuberculosis, 55, 168
Tumors, 166, 168. *See also* Organic
    affective disorder
Twins, 154

Unipolar depression, 86

Valium. *See* Diazepam

Valproic acid, 100
Vegetative symptoms: in depression,
    19-20; in mania, 82
Viruses, 168
Vivactil, 44. *See also* Antidepressant
    medications

Weight loss, 15-19, 25. *See also*
    Anorexia nervosa
Winter depression. *See* Seasonal
    affective disorder

Xanax. *See* Alprazolam